Trust and Integrity in Biomedical Research

Trust and Integrity in Biomedical Research

The Case of Financial Conflicts of Interest

Edited by

Thomas H. Murray and Josephine Johnston

THE HASTINGS CENTER, GARRISON, NEW YORK

The Johns Hopkins University Press

Baltimore

© 2010 The Johns Hopkins University Press
All rights reserved. Published 2010
Printed in the United States of America on acid-free paper
9 8 7 6 5 4 3 2 1

The Johns Hopkins University Press
2715 North Charles Street
Baltimore, Maryland 21218-4363
www.press.jhu.edu

Library of Congress Cataloging-in-Publication Data

Trust and integrity in biomedical research : the case of financial conflicts of
interest / edited by Thomas H. Murray and Josephine Johnston.
    p. ; cm.
  Includes bibliographical references and index.
  ISBN-13: 978-0-8018-9626-2 (hardcover : alk. paper)
  ISBN-10: 0-8018-9626-6 (hardcover : alk. paper)
  1. Medicine—Research—Finance—Moral and ethical aspects.   2. Conflict
of interests.   I. Murray, Thomas H., 1946–   II. Johnston, Josephine.
  [DNLM: 1. Biomedical Research—ethics.   2. Bioethical Issues.   3. Con-
flict of Interest—economics.   4. Financial Support—ethics.   5. Health Policy.
W 20.55.E7 T873 2010]
  R852.T78 2010
  610.72068'1—dc22   2009043788

A catalog record for this book is available from the British Library.

*Special discounts are available for bulk purchases of this book. For more information,
please contact Special Sales at 410-516-6936 or specialsales@press.jhu.edu.*

The Johns Hopkins University Press uses environmentally friendly book
materials, including recycled text paper that is composed of at least 30 percent
post-consumer waste, whenever possible. All of our book papers are acid-free,
and our jackets and covers are printed on paper with recycled content.

Contents

Preface

Over the past two decades, changes in the structure and financing of biomedical research have brought new opportunities for financial gain to investigators, universities, hospitals, medical centers, and other individuals and organizations in the biomedical research world. This financial gain has come in the form of fees for service, company stock, incentive payments, licensing revenue, research sponsorship, monetary and equipment donations, and positions of influence on company management and advisory boards. The most recent comprehensive analysis of biomedical research funding found that by 2003, industry funded approximately 57 percent of U.S. biomedical research and development, compared with 32 percent in 1980 (Moses et al. 2005). A significant portion of this research takes place within universities, with between one-fifth and one-half of biomedical companies' research budgets spent on sponsoring research in academic institutions (Moses and Martin 2001). In addition to revenue from research sponsorship or contracts, universities and individual researchers are benefiting financially from changes in government policy encouraging them to patent the results of federally funded research.

During the same time period, stories in the media have raised public concern that these financial arrangements may be having a negative effect on the quality of research and on its usefulness for public policy. The most common concern is that these new financial arrangements create "conflicts of interest"—that is, conflicts between the obligation to conduct research according to scientific and ethical principles and the desire for financial gain. The fear is that these conflicts of interest will adversely affect the quality of research, causing harm to human research subjects and creating a body of research results that are at best unreliable and at worst misleading—and that trust in and support for biomedical research will erode. Although these

conflicts of interest occur throughout the biomedical research world, the relationships that most often attract concern are those between industry (particularly the pharmaceutical and medical device industries) and academia,
perhaps because academia has traditionally been viewed as pursuing knowledge for its own sake rather than for financial gain. Recently, however, this
outrage has extended to relationships between, for example, for-profit research
management firms and community physicians, as well as between government scientists and industry.

One prominent example of the debate over financial conflicts of interest
involved scientists at the National Institutes of Health (NIH). Beginning in
December 2003, the *Los Angeles Times* published a series of articles detailing
financial relationships between senior NIH scientists and industry, including
profiles of several scientists who had received hundreds of thousands of dollars in consulting fees and other compensation during the past decade from
companies with an interest in NIH research (Willman 2003a, 2003b). Where
once the NIH was described as "an island of objective and pristine research,
untainted by the influences of commercialization" (Willman 2003b, A1), the
Times's revelations questioned the objectivity and commitment to the public
good of at least some scientists working at the NIH. In response to these allegations, both the NIH and the Office of Government Ethics launched investigations that led to changes in NIH policy, including a ban on senior NIH
employees' accepting consulting payments from drug companies (U.S. Department of Health and Human Services 2005).

Other examples of financial interests raising questions about research
quality and objectivity abound, and some are described in chapter 1 of this
book. In addition to these public controversies, a number of empirical studies
have been published in academic and professional journals over the past fifteen years that show correlations between investigators' financial interests
and research results that favor the interests of the research sponsor, as well as
between industry funding of research and increased delays in the publication
of research results and refusals to share data with colleagues (Bekelman, Li,
and Gross 2003). These and other empirical findings, together with general
academic scholarship, have created a body of literature expressing concern
that financial arrangements in biomedical research are adversely affecting
the quality of biomedical research, exposing human subjects to elevated research risk, increasing secrecy among scientists, delaying or preventing the
publication of research results, skewing the direction of research, and eroding public trust in both the biomedical research process and its results.

These concerns for the integrity of biomedical research motivated a Hastings Center project on ethical issues in the management of financial conflicts of interest in biomedical research, generously funded by the Patrick and Catherine Weldon Donaghue Medical Research Foundation. This book brings together contributions from members of the center's project working group, a diverse group of scholars and stakeholders who met and debated conflict-of-interest issues, along with additional invited experts.

The book begins with an overview of conflict of interest in biomedical research, followed by three chapters that consider different aspects of the broad context in which financial conflicts of interest emerge. In chapter 1, Josephine Johnston (one of the editors) describes how financial interests in biomedical research arise, who has them, why, and how (it is feared) they will affect research quality and trust. She describes how financial interests are thought to conflict with the goals of biomedical research and, through an exploration of the importance of trust in biomedical research, explains why the financial interests of certain players in the biomedical research system receive so much attention. Johnston argues that the prevalence of financial interests, correlations between financial interests and pro-sponsor results and increased secrecy, and a common understanding of the potential for money to bias judgment, taken together, mean that financial interests can threaten the quality and trustworthiness of biomedical research. Johnston explains that conflict-of-interest policies and rules aim to reduce the risk posed by conflicts of interest—they are a form of risk management—rather than to identify actual bias or other research misconduct. Because conflicts of interest pose only a risk, not a certainty, of harm to the quality and trustworthiness of research, and because financial interests bring benefits, policies need to distinguish between those interests that will never be tolerated, those that will always be tolerated, and those that can be permitted only after following certain measures, such as further disclosure of the financial interest, addition of disinterested researchers to the team, or additional oversight. Johnston concludes by emphasizing the need for community "buy-in" for rules and policies to be effective. She also calls for attention to the funding landscape within which financial conflicts of interest arise in biomedical research.

In chapter 2, Neetika Prabhakar Cox, Christopher Heaney, and Robert M. Cook-Deegan focus on this funding context, highlighting those features that intensify conflicts between norms of Mertonian open science and commercial private research and development. They begin by reviewing facts and figures about health research in the period since World War II, and then turn to observations about the context in which issues of "conflict of interest" have been framed. They conclude that health research is now big science and also big business and predict that managing contending social goals and financial interests is going to be a prominent task at academic research institutions for the foreseeable future. They note that more and better data are essential to guide future policy and that transparency is only a necessary and not a sufficient condition for the long-term health of the system—a necessary condition that has not yet been achieved. In addition to information and openness, the authors call for credible norms and practices to ensure that research, particularly when it is publicly financed, achieves its intended social benefit.

Henry Etzkowitz, author of chapter 3, is also interested in the context in which financial conflicts of interest are generated. Etzkowitz traces the evolution of academic research in the United States and considers the pros and cons of its current emphasis on commercializing research. He focuses on the role that patenting and commercialization have played in the advancement of both individual research institutions and society as a whole, arguing that the overall gains for individuals, institutions, and society of academic-industry collaborations and academic patenting outweigh financial conflict-of-interest concerns.

In chapter 4, Eric G. Campbell, Darren E. Zinner, Greg Koski, and David Blumenthal present data on the nature, extent, and consequences of the "triple helix" of relationships between academia, government, and industry in the life and health-related sciences. They present what is currently known about the nature and extent of relationships between government and academic scientists and industry, before providing evidence supporting the benefits of these relationships for individual scientists, their institutions, and the advancement of science. They then discuss the potential risks of such relationships, outline current policies to supervise them, and provide a set of guiding principles and policy suggestions regarding the disclosure and management of relationships among the various sectors.

To gain some comparative wisdom, in part II of the book, we consider how other professions conceptualize and manage conflicts of interest. John R. Boatright begins by offering a detailed description of how financial conflicts of interest are managed in the financial services industry, which he characterizes as a risk-management strategy. Generally, the parties are free to negotiate which financial interests service providers will be permitted to hold. Contracts, therefore, rather than federal policies play a large part in the management of financial interests. Boatright concludes with a set of six lessons from financial services, which can help in formulating policy in other areas; these include suggestions that parties be given sufficient flexibility to adapt policies to their individual circumstance and that parties not overlook compliance issues.

In chapter 6, law professor Robert Lawry traces the development of professional standards for lawyers that deal with conflicts of interest, from the 1908 Canon of Professional Ethics up to the American Bar Association's Model Rules of Professional Conduct. He notes the change from ethics rules, which focused on setting standards of good professional conduct, to laws and law-like rules, which establish standards below which lawyers may not fall. Lawry also observes a move from "risk rules," which aim to avoid situations in which a lawyer's judgment is at risk, to "harm rules," which aim to remedy actual harm caused by impaired judgment—a change that tends to permit more conflicts of interest, provided that certain procedures are followed, including disclosing the conflict, obtaining informed consent, and creating "screens" or walls between lawyers within firms. Lawry considers lawyers' two main conflicts of interest, conflicts with current clients and conflicts with previous clients, and describes how the rules dealing with those conflicts have changed over time, ultimately leading to the acceptance of far more conflicts of interest than was traditionally the case in the legal profession.

Rounding out our consideration of how other professions understand and respond to conflicts of interest, in chapter 7, journalism professor Deni Elliott argues that journalists might have the broadest definition of a conflict of interest and some of the strictest norms and institutional rules dealing with the issue. As Elliott explains, however, journalism is not united in the same way as are some licensed professions, norms of impartiality are under challenge as news organizations merge with entertainment, and institutional conflicts of interest have become more common. Elliott describes the scope of conflicts that impede, or can be perceived as impeding, journalists from doing their jobs and explains why the mere appearance of a conflict of interest matters to journalists and their news-organization employers. She reviews a sampling of individual conflicts and describes some representative organizational conflicts, explaining both why those conflicts are of concern to journalism and what is being done to address them. Her chapter ends with a consideration of how the expansion of reporting platforms to include the internet and its cadre of citizen-journalists raises new questions for journalism and requires ongoing diligence.

Law professor William M. Sage closes this part of the book by comparing the meaning of conflict of interest in law with the use made of the term in biomedical research. He notes that criticism of financial relationships in biomedical research has been widespread, with individuals, organizations, associations, and government entities universally labeling such relationships "conflicts of interest." Yet he finds the term vague, tending to mix specific relational obligations to patients with general ideals of purity that are challenged not only by commercialism but also by other human frailties. Sage argues that a conflict-of-interest framework is inappropriate for protecting the purity of biomedical research, which would be better achieved through a framework that focused on managing financial incentives. His goal is to challenge the legal and ethical language of the current response and the implications of that language—not the underlying need for current action or future vigilance.

In part III, we include a chapter describing current responses to financial conflicts of interest in biomedical research and a chapter that details the experience of this debate from the perspective of contract research organizations, which are sometimes accused of exacerbating the problem. Increased attention to conflicts of interest by government agencies, Congress, professional societies, and the public has resulted in many academic institutions developing or revising their policies, procedures, and practices for managing conflicts of interest. In chapter 9, David Perlman discusses the current regulatory regime and ethical, policy, and operational considerations that institutions might wish to consider for developing or revising policies to manage financial conflicts of interest in biomedical research. First, he highlights some recent events that have prompted increased scrutiny in conflicts of interest and how this increased scrutiny affects compliance efforts and public trust in the research enterprise. Next, to assist institutions that undertake the task of revising or developing conflict-of-interest policies and procedures in light of recent reports and guidance documents, he provides a detailed comparison of the current regulations with several of these reports and guidance documents. Perlman's aim is to help institutions consider several key policy elements that will bolster public trust in the research enterprise through proactive and effective management of financial conflicts of interest.

Contract research organizations (CROs) are commercial companies that contract with pharmaceutical, biotechnology, and medical device companies to run clinical trials. CROs employ more than seventy thousand people worldwide and conduct thousands of clinical trials in more than sixty countries. In this final chapter, Douglas Peddicord, legislative director of the Association of

Clinical Research Organizations, responds to the allegation that CROs are more likely to create and experience financial conflicts of interest than nonprofit participants in clinical research, arguing that financial and regulatory pressures on CROs provide strong incentives for avoiding damaging financial interests.

If it was once the case that biomedical researchers, particularly those working for nonprofit institutions, avoided acquiring financial interests in biomedical research and considered relationships with industry to be contaminating, this is no longer the rule. Financial conflicts of interest are now common among individuals and institutions involved in biomedical research. This prevalence suggests that individuals and institutions in biomedical research either do not understand, or do not believe, that these interests carry risks, that they believe themselves to be adequately managing these risks already, or that they believe avoidance and/or management is not possible or desirable.

While there is little definitive evidence that financial interests are impairing judgment or causing a loss of public trust, we do have data showing a correlation between financial interests and both pro-sponsor research and increased secrecy, as well as examples of significant media and political concern about the financial interests of individuals involved in academic and government research. In addition, the idea that financial interests can threaten the quality of research has strong intuitive appeal. These data and these intuitions, as well as comparisons with professions that take conflict-of-interest management seriously, together form the basis for the concern that financial conflicts of interest threaten the quality and trustworthiness of biomedical research.

Until more data exist, it may not be possible to convince everyone that financial conflicts of interest are anything more than a public relations problem. As Bekelman, Li, and Gross (2003, 45) commented, "consensus for reform may only arise from a full understanding of the nature and influence of financial conflicts of interest." Nevertheless, regular media attention and continued expressions of concern in scholarly and professional writing suggest that many commentators from both outside and inside the biomedical research community believe that financial conflicts of interest threaten the quality and trustworthiness of research and that whatever is currently being done is not sufficient to manage these risks.

Most commentators remain committed to self-regulation within the biomedical research community (i.e., committed to institutions, organizations, funders, and journals setting rules for the avoidance and management of financial interests). Similarly, most commentators and most policies continue to rely on investigators' honesty, particularly during initial disclosure. Unfortunately, many conflict-of-interest policies are complex, difficult to navigate, and less than adequately enforced. If investigators, research institutions, and research regulators continue to hold financial interests in their research and continue to fail to institute, enforce, and comply with policies requiring the management of these interests, it may become necessary to abandon either the goal of impartiality or the commitment to self-regulation.

To avoid the development of radically different policies, including bans or external management, new policies should be developed to cover institutional financial conflicts of interest, and existing policies on individual financial conflicts of interest should be, at a minimum, simplified, unified, routinely reassessed, and properly enforced. In particular, policies should clearly and reasonably differentiate between those conflicts of interest that are impermissible and therefore must be avoided altogether and those that can be accommodated, provided that other measures are taken. For the policies to work, they must be supplemented by education and awareness-raising to strengthen understanding of and support for conflict-of-interest management by those who must follow and enforce the policies. Those who must trust the research (research subjects, patients, health care professionals, policymakers, and so forth) should not be expected to do so "blindly" but should have good reasons to believe that financial interests will not exert an inappropriate influence over the judgment of those involved in the conduct, oversight, and assessment of that research. Concurrent research should continue to gather data on the feared risks of damage to the quality and trustworthiness of research, as well as on the cultural barriers to implementing and enforcing conflict-of-interest management policies.

Barriers to improvement are probably many, but an important one is the mixed messages on the propriety of financial interests. Individuals and institutions witness the outcry that often accompanies revelations of financial conflicts of interest (with or without accompanying problems with research quality). But technology transfer and receipt of industry research funds are also encouraged and expected, including by the federal government, and often carry significant financial and other benefits. As long as mixed messages about the propriety of financial interests and a lack of data persist, cultural change may be extremely difficult. There is no simple solution to this problem. Institutions, policymakers, and professional organizations will need to acknowledge the benefits and risks of the relationships that generate financial conflicts of interest and the care required to navigate them. A sympathetic response to the bind that some institutions and individuals feel themselves to be in—including an acknowledgment that financial conflicts of interest will occur—and the provision of tools for avoiding or managing financial interests will surely prove more useful than condemnation or a cavalier disregard.

Finally, continued discussion of the relationship between incentives in research, funding, and financial conflicts of interest is important. As much as possible, this discussion should reach outside the biomedical community. Institutional and individual financial conflict-of-interest management runs the risk of being seen simply as "window dressing"—a way to make any conflicts of interest appear innocuous, without the institution or individual forgoing its financial stake. Addressing this risk in public communication will be challenging.

REFERENCES

Bekelman, J. E., Y. Li, and C. P. Gross. 2003. Scope and impact of financial conflicts of interest in biomedical research: A systematic review. *JAMA* 289 (4): 454–65.

Moses, H., III, E. R. Dorsey, D. H. M. Matheson, and S. O. Thier. 2005. Financial anatomy of biomedical research. *JAMA* 294 (11): 1333–42.

Moses, H., III, and J. B. Matheson. 2001. Academic relationships with industry: A new model for biomedical research. *JAMA* 285 (7): 933–35.

U.S. Department of Health and Human Services. 2005. Supplemental standards of ethical conduct and financial disclosure requirements for employees of the Department of Health and Human Services. 5 CFR Parts 5501 and 5502. *Federal Register* 70 (168): 51559–74.

Willman, D. 2003a. Records of payments to NIH staff sought. *Los Angeles Times*, Dec. 9.

———. 2003b. Stealth merger: Drug companies and government medical research. *Los Angeles Times*, Dec. 7.

Contributors

David Blumenthal, M.D., M.P.P., is National Coordinator for Health Information Technology, U.S. Department of Health and Human Services.

John R. Boatright, Ph.D., is Professor of Ethics at Loyola University Chicago's Graduate School of Business, Illinois.

Eric G. Campbell, Ph.D., is Assistant Professor at the Institute for Health Policy, Massachusetts General Hospital–Partners Health Care System and Harvard Medical School, Boston, Massachusetts.

Robert M. Cook-Deegan, M.D., is Director of the Center for Genome, Ethics, Law and Policy at Duke University, Durham, North Carolina.

Neetika Prabhakar Cox, M.P.P., is an independent policy consultant, New York, New York.

Deni Elliott, Ph.D., is Professor in the Department of Journalism and Media Studies, University of South Florida, St. Petersburg, Florida.

Henry Etzkowitz, Ph.D., is Visiting Professor, Edinburgh University Business School, and Faculty Research Fellow, Clayman Institute for Gender Research, Stanford University, Stanford, California.

Christopher Heaney, B.A., is Research Aide at the Center for Genome, Ethics, Law and Policy at Duke University, Durham, North Carolina.

Josephine Johnston, L.L.B., M.B.H.L., is Research Scholar at The Hastings Center, Garrison, New York.

Greg Koski, Ph.D., M.D., is Senior Scientist at the Institute for Health Policy, Massachusetts General Hospital–Partners Health Care System and Harvard Medical School, Boston, Massachusetts.

Robert Lawry, J.D., L.L.M., is Professor Emeritus and Director of the Center for Professional Ethics at Case Western Reserve University School of Law, Cleveland, Ohio.

Thomas H. Murray, Ph.D., is President of The Hastings Center, Garrison, New York.

Douglas Peddicord, Ph.D., is Executive Director of the Association of Clinical Research Organizations, Washington, DC.

David Perlman, Ph.D., is Senior Lecturer at the University of Pennsylvania School of Nursing, Philadelphia, Pennsylvania.

William M. Sage, M.D., J.D., is Vice Provost for Health Affairs at the University of Texas at Austin, Texas.

Darren E. Zinner, Ph.D., is Senior Research Associate at the Health Industry Forum at Brandeis University, Waltham, Massachusetts.

PART I

MEANING AND CONTEXT

CHAPTER 1

Financial Conflicts of Interest in Biomedical Research

JOSEPHINE JOHNSTON, L.L.B., M.B.H.L.

Substantial time and money are devoted to biomedical research. Based on this research, thousands of drugs and medical devices are approved, millions of prescriptions are written, patients undergo numerous procedures and make significant health-related decisions, governments and other funders decide how to allocate billions of precious research dollars, and new biomedical research is conducted.

One of the consequences of these countless decisions is an increase in knowledge of human health and disease. Indeed, the promise of more knowledge encourages governments, companies, charitable groups, and members of the public to support biomedical research—financially, politically, and personally (for example, by enrolling in clinical trials). Because so many rely on biomedical research and because it affects human health, threats to its quality and trustworthiness are generally taken seriously, not only by those within the biomedical research system but also by policymakers and members of the public. One of these threats, conflicting financial interests, is the subject of this book.

Over the past few decades, the medical and biological sciences literature has increasingly expressed the concern that individual and institutional commitment to conducting, overseeing, and assessing biomedical research according to scientific and ethical standards might waver if these individuals or institutions could financially benefit or suffer a loss, depending on the outcome of the research. The fear is that if financial interests prove inconsistent with research-related obligations, institutions or individuals might consciously—or unconsciously—favor these interests, thereby generating flawed research. Even if their judgment is not, in fact, tainted, research conducted, overseen, or assessed by those with financial conflicts of interest risks appearing untrustworthy.

In recent years, individual researchers, institutions, journals, professional societies, industry, and the federal government have taken various steps to deal with financial conflicts of interest. Managing such conflicts has not been easy for any of those involved, and it is not clear whether the measures thus far adopted have protected research quality or trust. Despite reform efforts, financial conflicts of interest persist in both clinical and nonclinical biomedical research. In fact, much of this reform has allowed the retention of financial interests, opting instead for disclosure and other measures aimed at reducing the risk of harm. Reluctance to eliminate financial interests altogether may be due to the benefits such interests bring to both individuals and institutions. The flip side of these benefits, however, is that financial interests continue to stir up disagreements and controversies.

In this chapter, I seek to lay out a number of issues, as clearly as possible, at two main levels of analysis. The first includes big-picture and conceptual issues such as how financial interests in biomedical research arise, who holds these interests and why, how the interests might affect research quality and trust, and what benefits they seem to offer. The second level includes practical issues such as what is currently being done about financial conflicts of interest in biomedical research and what needs to be done better. I do not devote much attention to details such as the precise dollar value of disclosure thresholds or the specific components of conflict-of-interest education. This third level of analysis, while important, is more properly addressed by professional organizations, regulators, and individual institutions.

The Goals of Biomedical Research and the Nature of Financial Interests

Biomedical research is scientific research "pertaining to those aspects of the natural sciences, especially the biologic and physiological sciences, that relate to or underlie medicine" (Medical Economics Company 1995, 205). The core purpose of biomedical research, therefore, is the generation of new knowledge related to medicine. Particular projects may or may not involve human subjects.

The individuals involved in the conduct, oversight, and assessment of biomedical research usually work in one of three kinds of institution: (1) non-profit institutions, including universities, medical schools, hospitals, and professional organizations such as the American Academy for the Advancement of Science (which publishes the journal *Science*) and the American Medical Association (which publishes *JAMA*, the *Journal of the American Medical Association*); (2) the federal government, including agencies that conduct and fund biomedical research, such as the National Institutes of Health (NIH), or that rely on this research when making regulatory decisions, such as the Food and Drug Administration (FDA); and (3) commercial entities such as pharmaceutical companies, commercial research organizations, and commercial publishers (for example, the company that publishes the *Nature* journals).

Within these institutions, the individuals involved in biomedical research vary greatly in the type of work they do. They may be bench or clinical scientists; physicians, nurses, or other medical professionals; students; journal editors; members of institutional review boards (IRBs) or conflict-of-interest committees; or administrators such as CEOs or university presidents, grant officers, managers, or bureaucrats.

Most of these individuals must, at times, rely on their judgment. The conduct, oversight, and assessment of biomedical research are not simply mechanical activities. They frequently involve judgments about, for example, trial design, the suitability of particular research subjects, the balance of risk, or the balance of evidence. Many individuals who must exercise judgment also have the opportunity to hold financial interests in, or related to, the very research they are conducting, overseeing, or assessing, as do the institutions for which they work. The *potential* influence of these financial interests on the exercise of judgment raises concern.

A broad understanding of financial interests encompasses any financial relationship one person or organization has to another person or organization. The relationship could result from a recurrent payment such as a licensing fee or from a one-off payment such as a research grant, honorarium, contractual fee, or gift. It could have a range of monetary values, from very small to extremely large, and that value may be fixed or have the ability to increase or decrease (a patented invention, for example, has no fixed value and may be licensed for varying sums during the life of the patent). A financial interest may have a current value (e.g., cash or equipment), or the value may not yet be known or realizable (e.g., equity in new companies). Both individuals and institutions can hold financial interests.

Despite this wide range of financial interests and of individuals and institutions that can hold these interests, empirical research and commentary have generally focused on the financial interests of what I will call "noncommercial" institutions and individuals, particularly universities and their employees, federal agencies and their employees, members of federal advisory committees, and members of IRBs. Within this group, the financial interests of individuals (particularly academic scientists) have received considerably more attention than those of institutions, although concern is growing that institutions' financial stakes in research conducted by their staff and/or on their premises can conflict with their obligations to oversee that research and to operate in accordance with their missions (Association of American Universities 2001; AAMC Task Force on Financial Conflicts of Interest in Clinical Research 2002; U.S. General Accounting Office 2001; Institute of Medicine 2009).

New Financial Interests in Academic and Government Biomedical Research

Biomedical research has long been a money-making venture for companies and for some individual inventors. But traditionally, academic institutions and their employees have focused on their missions of teaching, research, and public service (including sometimes generating local growth) rather than on generating revenue through commercial activities. Likewise, U.S. government agencies and their employees have been distinguished from companies and their employees by a commitment to public service rather than to shareholders or investors (noticing such distinctions is not to suggest that these commitments are mutually exclusive but simply to compare priorities). These previously noncommercial individuals and institutions now have new and additional opportunities to make money, both from research contracts and other relationships with biomedical industries, particularly pharmaceutical and biotechnology companies, and from the commercialization of their own research. The contemporary debate about financial conflicts of interest and their management must be understood in this new context.

Knowledge generated within universities has always been transferred to private industry by graduating students, publications, and presentations (Rosenberg and Nelson 1994). Until a few decades ago, however, academic and government research institutions and their employees were not typically involved in the commercialization of their research. The 1980 Bayh-Dole Act states that institutions receiving federal funds may elect to patent any invention resulting from a federal grant, contract, or cooperative agreement (35 United States Code [USC] Sec. 200–212). That same year, Congress gave government agencies the power to patent the results of their in-house research (Stevenson-Wydler Technology Innovation Act of 1980; Federal Technology Transfer Act of 1986). In the six years from 2003 through 2008, the NIH alone was awarded an average of 95 U.S. patents per year (Office of Technology Transfer and National Institutes of Health 2008). Patents awarded to U.S. academic institutions quadrupled between 1995 and 2002, peaking at just under 3,300 patents issued per year, with one-third of all utility patents issued in the United States going to academic institutions (National Science Board 2008).

The 1980 law change played an important role in the growth of academic technology transfer activities. Technology transfer offices are now found in most academic research institutions. These offices patent and license inventions created at the institution by staff members (in 2007, U.S. universities earned more than $2 billion in license fees, options, and running royalties [Tieckelmann, Kordal, and Bostrom 2008]) and negotiate transfer of the inventions to outside researchers and companies, often in exchange for a license fee, equity in a "start-up" company (Stevens, Toneguzzo, and Bostrom 2005), or sponsorship of further research at the institution (Bekelman, Li, and Gross 2003).

During the same period that the Bayh-Dole Act encouraged academic institutions and government agencies to engage with industry, industry turned to academic institutions and their employees, not just for access to their intellectual property, but for individual expertise and as a venue for sponsored research. This latter activity provides institutions with funds, researchers with research opportunities, and industry with skilled investigators and respected sites for research. By the early twenty-first century, industry had become the largest source of funding for biomedical research, funding between 57 and 61 percent of clinical and nonclinical research (Moses et al. 2005; Institute of Medicine 2009) and spending between one-fifth and one-half of companies' research and development budgets in universities (Moses and Martin 2001).

Companies work with individual researchers at academic institutions and, until recently, researchers in government labs, whose knowledge, experience, and reputation can benefit companies seeking scientific advisors, educational speakers, and other consultants. Studies suggest that about one-fourth of academic biomedical researchers receive industry funding and that one-third of academic researchers and 60 percent of medical school department chairs have personal financial ties with industry (Bekelman, Li, and Gross 2003; Campbell et al. 2007).

Both these activities—the commercialization of in-house research and individual engagement with industry—are often welcomed by institutions and individuals for the professional and financial opportunities they create. Yet they also attract concern and generate controversy, because the resultant financial interests are considered to conflict with individuals' and institutions' research-related interests and obligations (Krimsky 2003). Conflict-of-interest policies have been developed in response to mixed messages about the propriety and value of these financial interests, and those policies are being implemented in this difficult context today.

Concerns about Financial Interests in Biomedical Research

As more of those involved in biomedical research have begun to hold financial interests in that research, journalists, scholars, and other commentators have raised the concern that these financial arrangements are creating "conflicts of interest" between, on the one hand, the obligation to conduct, oversee, and assess research according to scientific and ethical principles and, on the other hand, the desire for financial gain (Thompson 1993). The fear is that financial interests might adversely affect the *quality* of research, possibly harming human research subjects and anyone who later relies on the research, and the *appearance* of objectivity in that research. Financial interests are considered a threat or a risk, and financial conflict-of-interest policies are therefore about risk management; they are not about the identification of *bias*, which is covered by other policies and rules, but instead aim to identify and eliminate *risks* before those risks can lead to bias, other research misconduct, or a loss of trust.

While many in society can reap the rewards of biomedical research, few can assess the research for themselves. Patients and their physicians cannot usually critique the research that supports the use of a particular medication for a given condition. Journal editors rely on the opinion of peer reviewers, who themselves cannot always completely assess a study from the information they receive (Kennedy 2006). Even other biomedical researchers, who may well understand their colleagues' work, do not generally have the time or the resources to repeat it. Instead, almost everyone who uses biomedical research must, at least to some extent, *trust* that it is accurate and reliable. It is no exaggeration to say that trust is essential in the current system of biomedical research.

Yet trust can be lost, either as a result of negative experiences and evidence (e.g., studies reporting links between financial interests and flawed research) or because of suspicion and supposition. Even though it can seldom, if ever, be proved that financial interests have *caused* actors to waver in their commitment to biomedical research, and even though it is contested *which financial interests* might inappropriately influence *which actors* and under *what circumstances*, the suspicion that money can influence action—and particularly that it can exert an inappropriate influence—seems to be widely held. This suspicion threatens to undermine trust in the results of biomedical research as well as in biomedical researchers, their institutions, and the whole biomedical research system.

Indeed, over the past decade, the media, politicians, and other commentators have reacted strongly to reports of financial interests in biomedical research, both where specific problems with that research have surfaced *and* where no problems are apparent. After nineteen-year-old Jesse Gelsinger died in a University of Pennsylvania gene transfer study in 1999, conflicts of interest were among the allegations leveled at the research team and the university. The *Washington Post* reported that both the university and the lead investigator held equity stakes in a company with a financial interest in the vector used in the experiment and that the lead investigator and medical school dean held patents on processes used in the trial (Nelson and Weiss 2000). Although no causal relationship could be established between these financial interests and the irregularities associated with Gelsinger's death, the presence of financial interests raised the suspicion that concern for financial gain clouded the judgment of those involved in the trial.

In another often-cited case, the *Los Angeles Times* reported in 1998 that more than half the scientists involved in the testing of Rezulin, a drug for treatment of type II diabetes, had received research funding or compensation from the manufacturer. The drug was fast-tracked through the FDA approval process on the basis of these scientists' research, but its approval was cancelled three years later when it was shown that the drug led to liver failure in at least ninety patients. The concern expressed in newspaper reports and in subsequent academic commentaries was that scientists involved in assessing Rezulin who also had a financial interest in the drug's success may have reviewed the drug more positively than the evidence warranted (Krimsky 2003).

Similar controversies continue to emerge. In February 2005, a FDA advisory panel voted to continue to allow sale of the COX-2 inhibitors Celebrex, Bextra, and Vioxx. A week later, the *New York Times* reported that ten of the thirty-two panel members had recently been consultants to the manufacturers of the drugs, leading to the speculation that if these conflicted researchers had been left off the panel, two of the three drugs would have been withdrawn from the market (Harris and Berenson 2005).

In late 2004 and early 2005, the *Los Angeles Times* published a series of articles detailing financial relationships between senior NIH scientists and industry (Knight 2003; Willman 2003a, 2003b). No problems with the research or administrative work of the scientists were reported. Nevertheless, where once the NIH was described as "an island of objective and pristine research, untainted by the influences of commercialization" (Willman 2003b, A1), revelations that some NIH staff collected hundreds of thousands of dollars under consultancy and other arrangements from companies whose products were the subject of intra- or extramural research and that the NIH failed to require disclosure of such interests to human research subjects were enough to lead some commentators and politicians to question the institutes' objectivity and commitment to public health (Willman 2003a, 2003b; Johnston 2004; Steinbrook 2004).

In 2008, several conflict-of-interest stories were reported in major U.S. newspapers, a number of which were prompted by ongoing investigations by Senator Charles Grassley of Iowa. One *New York Times* cover story reported alleged failures by psychiatrists at Massachusetts General Hospital to disclose tens of thousands of dollars in income received from drug companies. The most dramatic allegations were against child psychiatrist Joseph Biederman, who, as the *Times* reported, had received more than $1.6 million in payments from drug companies between 2000 and 2007 but had reported little of that income to his institution. The allegations against Biederman were aggravated by his prominent support for expanding the diagnosis of bipolar disorder among children and its treatment with medications (Harris and Carey 2008).

In addition to these public controversies, empirical studies conducted over the past two decades have fueled concern. Some studies simply documented the prevalence of financial interests among individuals and institutions involved in biomedical research. For example, a 2003 review article found ten studies reporting that between 23 and 28 percent of individual academic investigators received research funding from industry, more than 40 percent received research-related gifts, and "approximately one third of investigators at academic institutions have personal financial ties with industry sponsors" (Bekelman, Li, and Gross 2003, 456). The 1999 Association of University Technology Managers (AUTM) survey found that 68 percent of responding institutions held equity in companies that, in turn, sponsored research at that institution. An AUTM survey in 2003 reported that nearly 85 percent of institutions received research support linked to agreements to license or option technology that was or might be generated at the university (Stevens and Toneguzzo 2004), providing the university with a current or future financial interest in the work of its researchers. Other studies have documented correlations between industry funding of academic clinical research and pro-sponsor results, as well as between industry funding and increased secrecy, whether in the form of delays in publication of research results or refusals to share data with colleagues (Bekelman, Li, and Gross 2003).

These and other empirical findings, together with academic scholarship (Thompson 1993; Angell 2000; Krimsky 2003) and trade and magazine publications (Press and Washburn 2000; Bok 2003; Washburn 2005), have created a body of literature expressing the fear that many of the financial arrangements now common in biomedical research are damaging its quality and undermining its trustworthiness.

Primary Interests and Biomedical Research

For financial interests to be problematic, they must conflict with other, more important interests and obligations—with what I call here "primary interests." According to the definition quoted above, the primary goal of biomedical research is the generation of new knowledge about medicine (Merton 1973 [1942], 267–78; Campbell et al. 2005). In addition, because the latter half of the twentieth century saw a growth in concern for human research subjects, there is a strong argument that research subjects' health and well-being is also of primary importance in biomedical research (see 45 Code of Federal Regulations [CFR] Sec. 46.101–46.124; World Medical Association 2008). As a consequence, one can argue that the primary interests of all individuals and institutions that are conducting, assessing, and overseeing biomedical research ought to be the generation of new biomedical knowledge in a manner consistent with the rights and interests of any human research subjects (not all biomedical research involves human subjects) (Institute of Medicine 2009).

But it is unlikely that these are the *only* primary interests of every individual and institution involved in biomedical research. (To denote an interest as primary is not merely descriptive; it is also a normative statement about what should be the goal of the research and the major concern of everyone involved.) For one thing, the suggestion that they are the only primary interests is unrealistic. Some individuals and institutions involved in biomedical research can and should hold additional primary interests, including financial interests in satisfying clients or generating profits for shareholders. The financial interests of pharmaceutical or biotechnology companies, their employees, and their contractors are not and, arguably, should not be subordinate to their research-related interests: generating new biomedical knowledge and generating profits are transparently at the very heart of the industries' existence and are inherent in their role in the biomedical research system. Indeed, their financial interests attract little outside attention. The presence in the biomedical research system of checks and balances overseen by disinterested parties is one reason for this lack of concern. When a pharmaceutical company seeks FDA approval of a new drug, for instance, its financial interest in the research it has conducted and sponsored is, arguably, blunted by the FDA review process, which is supposed to root out any problems through unbiased expert review.

The biomedical research system is structured to accommodate some financial conflicts of interest, but not others. While financial interests are expected and tolerated in some roles, particular individuals and particular institutions are currently expected or required to be impartial and disinterested. Academic and government individuals and institutions have long played this role, whether as members of FDA committees, grant and article peer reviewers, researchers, or research sites, and many continue to hold themselves out as such, making them a focus of the conflict-of-interest debate (Campbell, Koski, and Blumenthal 2004).

Definition of Financial Conflicts of Interest

In the context considered here, an institution or individual will have a financial conflict of interest if it or he or she meets the following criteria:

1. Involvement in the conduct, oversight, or assessment of biomedical research; and
2. Having a financial interest that *might reasonably* be affected by that same biomedical research; and
3. Being under an expectation of impartiality (Davis and Stark 2001).

Determining criterion 1 is usually straightforward. Deciding whether someone meets criteria 2 and 3 can be difficult. Materiality (whether a financial interest counts for the purposes of establishing criterion 2) is complex. Appropriate proxies for an expectation of impartiality (criterion 3) may be non-profit status and/or involvement in the assessment of research (e.g., as a member of an FDA committee or the author of a review article), but application of this criterion will also be contested.

Conflict of interest is often confused with bias. Merely identifying a financial conflict of interest does not determine what its impact will be on a particular individual's or institution's judgment, nor does it mean that the individual or institution has necessarily committed a wrong (Institute of Medicine 2009). It simply means that the individual or institution is in a risky—and potentially controversial—situation, which must be examined and may require action. Conflict-of-interest rules and policies, therefore, aim to identify and manage risk, leaving the identification and management of bias or other research misconduct to other policies and rules.

Before proceeding, and in the light of William Sage's contribution to this volume (chapter 8), I should note that in this debate, the term *conflicts of interest* has a broader meaning than it often has in professional ethics (e.g., in the legal profession). Here, it retains its narrow, relational sense of a conflict between an individual's or institution's financial interests and specific obligations owed to identifiable individuals, but it also refers to a conflict between financial interests and interests or obligations that are not dependent on specific interpersonal relationships. We can meaningfully ask whether there is a conflict between an institution's obligation to the public to promote socially responsible research among its faculty and its financial interest in pursuing research from which it could gain financially, or between a research investigator's interest in patenting his invention and his obligation to the scientific community to promptly share his research findings. Sage disagrees with this interpretation and argues, persuasively, that these arrangements would more properly be considered to raise incentive problems than conflicts of interest (Sage 2007). In the end, however, the same core questions remain: which interests threaten research quality and trust and what can be done to address them?

Risks versus Benefits
The Threat to Trust

Because so much research-related activity involves judgment, it necessarily involves risk and uncertainty. Those who use the results of biomedical research must sometimes act on trust. This trust can be based on personal knowledge of the good character of the individual or institution in question or on the belief that he, she, or it shares a commitment to advancing knowledge. But trust need not rest solely on individual characteristics.

The biomedical research system includes norms, practices, rules, and laws that act as constraints on behavior and provide incentives for actors to remain committed to its primary interests. Informal constraints, such as competition and reputation and their ensuing norms and practices, while not codified or formally agreed upon, powerfully encourage or discourage particular behaviors. In addition, formal constraints, such as institutional rules or federal and state laws, also encourage some behaviors and discourage others (Hardin 2002). Breaching these formal and informal constraints can risk sanction, such as lost relationships, damaged reputation, lost funding, or a fine.

According to this theory of trust, individuals and institutions involved in biomedical research are trustworthy *both* because of their personal or institutional commitment to the primary interests of biomedical research *and* because biomedical research takes place within a system of external constraints backed by sanctions that further encourage fidelity to the primary interests. Thus, individuals and institutions are strongly encouraged to privilege biomedical research's primary interests—the proper conduct, oversight, and assessment of biomedical research and the protection of human research subjects—over any competing interests, including financial gain. These constraints and the transparent threat of sanctions should also reassure all who use the outcomes of biomedical research that its culture, norms, formal rules, and laws support a strong commitment to producing new knowledge and protecting research subjects. In these ways, biomedical research's formal and informal constraints encourage trust because they protect the research's *actual* and *apparent* quality.

Yet, even in a system with strong incentives to remain committed to the primary interests, trust can be damaged or lost altogether. If those who must trust biomedical research no longer believe that their interest in its proper conduct, oversight, and assessment is sufficiently shared—if they come to believe that other interests, such as financial interests, are taking precedence—trust may be lost. It may also be lost if the external constraints are no longer considered robust enough or are not enforced.

The Threat to Norms and Practices

Changes to norms and practices are sometimes considered an indication that financial interests are adversely affecting the norms of biomedical research. One account of the norms of science was famously expressed by the sociologist Robert Merton in 1942 (Merton 1973). He listed four norms: universalism, communism, disinterestedness, and organized skepticism. One way of understanding these norms (and the practices, rules, and laws that follow from them) is as supportive of science's primary interest in generating new knowledge. (Merton did not address biomedical research's particular additional interest in the health and well-being of human research subjects.) That is, these norms and practices, and all that follow from them, are significant external constraints protecting the quality and trustworthiness of biomedical research.

In his book *Science in the Private Interest: Has the Lure of Profits Corrupted Biomedical Research?* philosopher Sheldon Krimsky (2003) expresses deep concern that financial interests are eroding Merton's norms. As evidence for this concern, he cites studies reporting a correlation between financial interests and increased secrecy in biomedical research. Krimsky points to studies showing that industry-sponsored faculty were more likely than other faculty to report delays in publication of their research results (Blumenthal et al. 1997) and that industry sponsors sometimes required investigators to keep information confidential for six months in order to file for a patent (Blumenthal et al. 1996). Two studies reported that participation in commercial activities such as patenting or start-up companies made an investigator significantly more likely to withhold data (Blumenthal et al. 1997; Campbell et al. 2002), while other studies showed that between 12 and 34 percent of academic researchers had been denied access to research results (Bekelman, Li, and Gross 2003). Krimsky (2003, 84) uses these data to argue that greater secrecy, refusals to exchange and share materials, and a pattern of delayed publication "suggest a new tolerance among academic scientists for commercializing first and sharing later." That is, Krimsky takes the data to be evidence of deterioration in the norms of communism (or communalism, as he rephrases it) and dis-interestedness.

The Threat to Research Quality

A breakdown in norms could certainly cause a breakdown in trust, but it is not in itself direct evidence that financial conflicts of interest are harming research quality. In fact, there is currently little evidence that financial interests are *causing* the generation of flawed knowledge or *causing* harm to research subjects. Causal evidence on this issue can be close to impossible to gather, because it would require intimate knowledge of the conscious or unconscious motivations of individual decision makers. Instead, studies show *associations*—between financial interests and practices that are thought to damage or slow biomedical research (as discussed above) and between financial interests and questionable study design or results that repeatedly favor the research sponsor (Davidson 1986; Rochon et al. 1994; Bero and Rennie 1996; Stelfox et al. 1998; Friedberg et al. 1999; Kjaergard and Als-Nielsen 2002). Associations, while not proving causation, can cause concern about research quality and can have a direct impact on trust.

As reported in a review article by Bekelman, Li, and Gross (2003, 463): "Strong and consistent evidence shows that industry-sponsored research tends to draw pro-industry conclusions. By combining data from articles examining 1140 studies, we found that industry-sponsored studies were significantly more likely to reach conclusions that were favorable to the sponsor than were non-industry studies." Studies have also found associations between financial interests in research and questionable trial design. In the same 2003 review, Bekelman and colleagues identified studies showing a greater likelihood of trials funded by for-profit organizations to use an inactive control, a tendency among industry-sponsored studies to use a higher dose of the industry-associated drug than of the comparator drug, and a tendency for industry-sponsored trials to use poorly absorbed comparator drugs. Such trial design makes it more likely that the sponsor's drug will perform better than comparator drugs, and therefore fails to offer a realistic measure of the drug's effectiveness or safety.

Some commentators have noted that there may be good explanations for some differences in outcome in industry-sponsored studies; for example, industry sponsors selectively fund research that is likely to yield favorable conclusions (Campbell et al. 2005; Institute of Medicine 2009). Questionable trial design could also be explained by incompetence or inexperience. But these associations between trial design and pro-industry findings could also be the result of a conscious or unconscious desire to produce a particular research result—one from which the researchers, their institution, or a research sponsor will benefit financially.

The association between financial interests and both a breakdown in some of the norms of science and an increased likelihood of pro-sponsor research outcomes *suggests* that financial interests are damaging the quality of some biomedical research. Put another way, the data support the claim that financial conflicts of interest threaten (pose a risk to) biomedical research's quality and therefore its trustworthiness. Although it is contested how significant a risk to biomedical research these financial conflicts of interest are (the answer probably depends on the particular circumstances of each case), one could conclude, based on this risk, that all conflicting financial interests should be eliminated. However, a number of benefits and competing values have thus far persuaded the federal government, many institutions, and many individuals that the complete elimination of conflicting financial interests from biomedical research is undesirable.

Benefits to Individuals and Institutions

Although financial conflicts of interest are seldom thought to be good for biomedical research, the benefits to individuals, institutions, and society of the relationships and arrangements that create these conflicting financial interests are acknowledged (AAMC Task Force on Financial Conflicts of Interest in Clinical Research 2001; Association of American Universities 2001; Campbell et al. 2005; Institute of Medicine 2009). Eliminating all—or many—financial conflicts of interest could mean forfeiting some of these benefits, a proposition likely to meet with considerable resistance.

Collaborations between academic and government researchers and industry are believed to have brought new health-related products to market (Stevens and Toneguzzo 2004; Stossel 2005). Indeed, a perceived lack of new technologies resulting from federally sponsored research was the impetus for the Bayh-Dole Act, and some influential commentators believe the act succeeded in this goal: a 2001 task force of the Association of American Universities (2001, i) noted that "transferring university-developed knowledge to the private sector fulfills one of the goals of federally funded research, by bringing the fruits of research to the benefit of society." A similar task force of the Association of American Medical Colleges (AAMC) made the same point: "At the crucial interface between innovation and development, researchers from academic medicine often play a critical role by conducting the early translational research that gives rise to new products, and by testing these novel products for safety and efficacy" (AAMC Task Force on Financial Conflicts of Interest in Clinical Research 2001, 3–4).

The AAMC Task Force (2001) also noted that interactions between academia and industry can have positive economic consequences for the regions in which universities are located. In his book *MIT and the Rise of the Entrepreneurial University*, Henry Etzkowitz (2002, 89) writes that as a result of the commercialization activities of Massachusetts Institute of Technology, a "regional pattern of science and technology-based economic growth was created that has been the subject of world-wide emulation." Evidence of the local economic impact of universities can also be seen in Silicon Valley near Stanford University in California and at Research Triangle near Duke University in North Carolina (Etzkowitz 2002).

Industry-academic interactions can also have a positive effect on institutions' finances. Although government still funds the majority of academic research, financial interactions with industry have boosted the research budgets of institutions, as have related gifts and sponsorships, royalty payments, and dividends and proceeds from the sale of companies. The 2007 AUTM Survey reported that U.S. universities received more than $2 billion in license fees, options, and running royalties (Tieckelmann, Kordal, and Bostrom 2008). Of the 157 responding institutions, 27 reported license income of more than $10 million, including 10 universities earning more than $50 million from licenses. This revenue is highly prized because institutions have considerable latitude in spending it; the Bayh-Dole Act directs only that it be spent on "scientific research or education" (35 USC 200–212).

Some discussions also emphasize the benefits of close collaboration with industry for individual researchers and their students, including the opportunity to access data, equipment, and materials not otherwise available and the satisfaction of seeing basic research translated into commercial products (Campbell, Koski, and Blumenthal 2004). Individuals can also benefit financially from royalties, consulting fees, company equity, and other forms of compensation, which in a competitive marketplace can assist institutions with recruitment and retention. Average academic salaries have barely improved in real value for more than thirty years (Thornton 2009), and the salaries of nonacademic scientists, health professionals, and engineers consistently exceed those of their academic colleagues. In each case, the gap appears to be widening (Hamermesh 2002). And, the events of 2008–9 aside, the increased cost of real estate since 1991 has far exceeded inflation in many parts of the United States, including in areas where several large research universities are based (U.S. Federal Housing Finance Agency 2009). Housing prices, low increases in the real value of academic salaries, and a growing gap between academic and nonacademic salaries may have increased the perceived need among academic researchers for supplementary income.

Not all the benefits listed above necessitate conflicting financial interests (Angell 2000). In theory, individuals and institutions could work with industry without payment, and institutions could run their technology transfer activities without aiming to profit but simply to cover costs. In 2000, Marcia Angell called the claim that universities' ties to industry are necessary for technology transfer "greatly exaggerated," arguing that the value of financial ties for moving technology into the marketplace greatly depends on the particular arrangement. Grants may be helpful, she noted, "but it is highly doubtful whether many of the other financial arrangements facilitate technology transfer or confer any other social benefit" (Angell 2000, 1517).

Yet there seems to be a strong reluctance to *donate* time, expertise, or resources, including inventions, to industry, even if taking compensation risks generating financial conflicts of interest. Some of this reluctance may stem from belief in, as Thomas Stossel (2005, 1064) put it, the "no conflict, no interest" principle, according to which a financial stake increases commitment and the chance of success. Reluctance may also be grounded in the belief that preventing individuals from profiting from their effort is unfair when that effort does not directly interfere with the performance of their regular duties, as may be the case when individuals are consultants to industry outside regular working hours (the counterargument, of course, is that financial conflicts of interest do interfere by compromising impartiality). Some restrictions on individuals and institutions might also be seen as intrusions on privacy and freedom of association and could risk contradicting the terms of the Bayh-Dole Act, which explicitly encourages commercialization activity by federally funded institutions and mandates that institutions share royalties with individual inventors.

Current Management, Problem Areas, and Future Directions

Given the threats to research quality, human subjects, and trust, a simple management strategy would be to institute a sweeping ban on conflicting financial interests. Given the perceived benefits, however, and the lack of clarity about the magnitude of the risks, one might propose allowing all conflicting financial interests. Although some have advocated for one or the other of these strategies, currently, neither is realistic (biomedical research as we know it would have to be drastically reorganized or downsized) or desirable (for example, we do not have sufficient data to conclude that all conflicting financial interests are so damaging to research quality and trust that all must be eliminated). There may be situations in which a ban is appropriate and situations in which no rules need apply, but there will also be many situations between these two extremes.

In recognition of this continuum, systems have been set up that attempt to preserve trust and protect research quality by *managing* financial interests in biomedical research, although many of these systems are not yet sufficient. Ideally, management systems would differentiate among kinds of financial conflicts of interest based on what is known or reasonably suspected about their risk to research quality and trust—banning some, permitting others outright, and permitting some in certain situations subject to one or more conditions (e.g., that the researcher withdraw from the human subjects phase of the research, that the interest be further disclosed, that additional oversight of the research be established). Management requires advance identification of financial interests that might generate a conflict so that they can be avoided, as well as contemporaneous identification through disclosure.

In crafting management policies, several questions arise. Whose financial interests should be reported and to whom? Which financial interests generate conflicts and how serious a risk do these conflicts pose to research quality and trust? What are the management options? Who decides and who enforces the rules? Over the past decade, many of these questions have been answered in regulations covering federally funded biomedical researchers and government employees, in the recommendations of various professional organizations, in institutional rules, in journal policies, and so forth (see 42 CFR Part 50, Subpart F, Sec. 50.601–50.607 [U.S. Public Health Service 1996]; 21 CFR Sec. 54.1–54.6 [U.S. Food and Drug Administration 1998]; Institute of Medicine 2009).

Largely due to the federal regulations, financial conflict-of-interest policies for individual researchers are now commonplace in academic biomedical research institutions. In a 2001 report, the U.S. General Accounting Office (GAO; now the Government Accountability Office) made several criticisms of the regulations and their application by academic institutions, including that they are not directly linked to regulations on human subjects protection, which means that information about a financial conflict of interest might not be conveyed to IRBs or used in protecting research subjects. In its limited survey, the GAO was also concerned that none of the universities had formal processes for verifying whether researchers had fully disclosed their financial interests and that divestiture of financial interests was an option seldom used. It recommended that the regulations be supplemented with best-practice guidelines.

The following year, the NIH reviewed conflict-of-interest policies of more than a hundred institutions and concluded that many policies were diffused, confusing, and expressed in unclear language (National Institutes of Health and Office of Extramural Research 2002). In 2004, the U.S. Department of Health and Human Services issued voluntary guidance for IRBs, research institutions, and investigators, recommending that IRBs consider whether financial interests might adversely affect the rights and welfare of human research subjects and whether disclosure to research subjects should be required (the guidance was limited to research involving human subjects). Although the draft version of the guidance had recommended against financially conflicted clinical investigators being directly engaged in aspects of clinical trails, the final version contains no such presumption. The guidance is explicitly nonbinding, and its impact on institutions, investigators, and IRBs is not yet known.

In addition to the regulations and guidance issued by the federal government, some influential organizations have issued reports recommending practices to promote and improve the management of individual and institutional financial conflicts of interest in the academic research environment. Prominent examples of these recommendations include those issued by the Association of American Universities (2001), the Association of American Medical Colleges (AAMC Task Force on Financial Conflicts of Interest in Clinical Research 2001, 2002), the American Society of Gene Therapy (2000), the American Society of Clinical Oncology (2003), the Federation of American Societies for Experimental Biology (2006), and, most recently, the Institute of Medicine (2009).

The recommendations of these and other bodies vary in detail, but all express deep concern about the risk that financial interests pose to the quality and trustworthiness of biomedical research. However, like the federal regulations, none of these recommendations seek to eliminate financial interests altogether. They opt instead for a system of management that, first, defines conflicting interests so that they may be avoided, then requires their disclosure when they are nonetheless present. Various other measures may be required following disclosure, depending on the type and size of the financial interest, the particular situation (whether the conflicted party is engaged in research, publication, or assessment, etc.) and whether patients or human subjects are involved. In particular, some recommendations call for a presumption against a financially conflicted researcher participating in human subjects research. The most recent recommendations, from the Institute of Medicine (2009), call for the U.S. government to create a public national registry of payments from pharmaceutical, medical device, and biotechnology companies and their foundations to physicians, biomedical researchers, and institutions, among others. A similar proposal is contained in the Physician Payments Sunshine Act, first introduced in the U.S. Senate in 2007.

Prestigious peer-reviewed journals have some power in the conflict-of-interest debate, because they serve as the preferred clearinghouse for much biomedical research—the success of careers and discoveries can depend on publication in peer-reviewed journals. They have used this power to require authors' disclosure of their individual financial interests and, in rare cases, to prevent financially conflicted authors from publishing in their pages. Many biomedical journals began requiring disclosure of financial interests to editors in the mid-1980s. Today, most, but still not all, journals require disclosures from all authors (Cooper et al. 2006; Ancker and Flanagin 2007). Once disclosed to the editors, information about financial interests may be shared with reviewers (Krimsky and Rothenberg 2001), the article may be published with all or some conflicts disclosed alongside, or the article may be disqualified from publication. While this last strategy is uncommon, some journals do reject articles on the basis of conflict of interest.

Until 2002, the *New England Journal of Medicine* would not publish review articles or editorials from authors with financial interests in any company or its competitor whose products were discussed in the article. However, the journal experienced growing difficulty finding unconflicted authors and became concerned that pharmaceutical companies might become the "chief source of information about new therapies" (Drazen and Curfman 2002, 1901). In testimony to the limits of this prestigious journal's powers, it revised its policy to exclude only those review authors with "significant" financial interests (personal interests valued at more than $10,000, or where profit is unlimited, and major research funding from relevant companies).

As noted above, in response to disclosures from authors, editors disclose some or all of an author's financial interests to readers. Disclosing to readers theoretically allows them to make an independent assessment of the article's quality and trustworthiness. One small study of *BMJ* readers' responses to an article in which a disclosure stated that the authors were employees of a pharmaceutical company reported a significant effect on perceptions of the scientific credibility of the articles, with readers finding financially conflicted reports "less interesting, important, relevant, valid and believable" (Chaudhry et al. 2002, 1391).

Yet, in real life, disclosure statements can be far harder for readers and editors to understand, because the link between disclosed interests and the research is not generally spelled out. An article describing a clinical trial might include a list of companies for whom one of the authors has consulted, but it may not be clear which company makes which drug or that one of the companies makes a competitor drug. For disclosure to be meaningful, therefore, the link between the interest and the research reported may need to be spelled out. But it may not be practical or particularly meaningful to publish long lists of conflicting interests alongside articles. And if conflicts become widespread, disclosure may no longer serve to alert readers.

Journals' disclosure policies reflect the belief that bias or partiality in research cannot always be detected simply through the peer review process and that preserving readers' trust involves some management of conflicts of interest. However, where management involves little more than choosing to further disclose selected financial interests to readers, it may do little to protect research quality or enhance trust (see the discussion of the limits of disclosure below). Journals can find themselves between a rock and a hard place, however, if more stringent policies make publication impractical or suitable authors impossible to find.

Existing management policies generally do not extend to institutional conflicts of interest and seem to be inadequately understood, followed, enforced, or assessed. The mixed messages that many individuals and institutions receive about the propriety of financial interests surely contribute to these problems, as does the reluctance of some researchers to be subject to management. Additional challenges arise in determining relevance, the best use of disclosure, and integration of conflict-of-interest committees and IRBs.

Determining which financial interests generate a conflict is complex. Which kinds of interest are sufficiently *related to* a given piece of biomedical research, which are *large* enough to warrant consideration, and which are *temporally close* enough to seriously threaten judgment or trustworthiness? As defined above, financial interests generate a conflict when they are in or related to the biomedical research in question (not if or when they actually exert an inappropriate influence). Some financial interests are easily identified as related to a particular piece of research, such as when an investigator holds a patent on the drug she is administering to human subjects in a clinical trial. However, the relevance of other financial interests is not as clear.

In addition, the size of the financial interest is often considered relevant in determining whether it poses a threat. Federal regulations place *de minimis* values on interests that must be disclosed and managed, but these limits are probably imposed more for practical than for principled reasons. Indeed, the U.S. Department of Health and Human Services (2001) has noted that numerical values such as those it employs do not reflect an established limit for what does and what does not pose a risk to judgment. Conflict-of-interest policies can also be limited to financial interests that are currently active or were active within the recent past, such as during the past five years. Like the size limit, a temporal limit is probably motivated by practical concerns as well as the (unsubstantiated but intuitively appealing) belief that financial interests from the distant past are unlikely to exert influence.

In the light of these issues, a wide understanding of materiality—proximity, size, and time—is the most prudent approach. Practically speaking, however, most management policies need to place some limits on what "counts" as a financial conflict of interest in need of management by excluding very small or very remote interests. Finding the appropriate balance between efficiency and comprehensiveness is difficult and may require periodic revision. Once relevant financial interests are described, management policies should, although few do, distinguish between those conflicts of interest that must be avoided or eliminated and those that can be managed in other ways; lawyers make this distinction, dividing conflicts of interest into "consentable" and "unconsentable" (Davis and Johnston 2009). This kind of distinction will mean that some opportunities for financial gain by individuals and institutions must be turned down because they would create unacceptable conflicts of interest.

Where financial conflicts have not been or need not be avoided, disclosure is the key first step in managing conflict of interest. Unfortunately, studies have shown frequent failure to disclose financial interests, and controversies continue to emerge over nondisclosure (Krimsky and Rothenberg 2001; Tanner 2006; Harris and Carey 2008). Even when disclosure is accurate and complete, disclosure alone—particularly initial disclosure to journal editors and conflict-of-interest committees—is unlikely to remove threats to research quality and trust. Instead, where the disclosed conflict is considered serious, the research may be rejected on account of the disclosed interest, as could be the case when conflicts of interest are disclosed to the FDA or to a journal. In less serious cases, further management will be required, including further disclosure of the interest, perhaps to research subjects, readers, or the general public. A 2003 survey of 674 responses from five groups of stakeholders (senior investigators, senior research administrators, bioethicists, journal editors, and agency administrators) reported support for expanded disclosure, including to IRBs, funders, and journal editors, with mixed support for increased disclosure to research subjects (Brody et al. 2003). Care must be taken, however, that further disclosure does not carry the implicit message that "otherwise problematic outside activities are permissible as long as they are publicly disclosed" (Glynn 2004). As already discussed in the context of journal policies, further disclosure also has the potential to be confusing and/or to place an unfair onus on those disclosed to (as could be the case when further disclosure is made to research subjects). It must be meaningful and likely to help the recipients of the disclosure to make more informed decisions.

Initial disclosure can also be followed by other kinds of management, including appointment of additional oversight for the research, such as might be provided by a data-management committee or the addition of an unconflicted investigator to the project. When disclosure is not sufficient, institutions or individuals could be required to divest themselves of the interest before proceeding with the research or could be removed from the activity in question (as when institutions adopt a presumption against conflicted investigators participating in human subjects research). How decision makers deal with the information disclosed to them does and should vary, depending on the nature and materiality of the conflict of interest and the particular activity the conflicted individual or institution is engaged in. What should not vary is the comprehensiveness and regularity of initial disclosures by all involved in biomedical research or the commitment of those assessing these disclosures to following through with further meaningful action.

One result of all the regulations, institutional rules, professional recommendations, and journal policies is that individual researchers need to be familiar with the many different policies. The reach and details of the rules, regulations, and recommendations often vary (Cho et al. 2000). This variation may reflect the fact that different rules on the management (including disclosure) of financial interests apply to different situations. However, it may also result from a lack of widely shared understandings about which kinds of financial interest generate conflicts in which circumstance. Variability can also impede compliance—which, according to empirical studies, is poor—and create confusion (Cho et al. 2000; Lipton, Boyd, and Bero 2004).

Other reasons for poor compliance might include less than strict enforcement or frequent relaxation of policies and rules. There are no significant data on levels of enforcement at academic institutions, but investigation of policies at the NIH, which may or may not be indicative of practices elsewhere, has shown incomplete enforcement of conflict-of-interest policies (U.S. Office of Government Ethics 2004). The fact that conflicts of interest are seldom reported to Public Health Service granting agencies, as is required under the regulations, may also indicate poor enforcement of the rules at the institutional level.

Enforcement might be improved if institutions and others were better able to detect noncompliance. Because current management systems rely on honest initial disclosure, noncompliance at the level of disclosure is unlikely to be detected unless reported by peers or other parties or following investigation by journalists or other interested parties (Harris and Carey 2008). To improve compliance, policies could include general principles as well as specific rules, so that the reasons for policies are clearer. Improved enforcement and stricter penalties may also encourage compliance, as could better education about the goals of conflict-of-interest management; individuals are more likely to comply with rules that they understand and, better still, support.

Culture and Education: Enabling Better Management

Comprehensively and effectively managing financial conflicts of interest in biomedical research is a complex task that takes time and uses precious resources. Policies need to be devised, assessed, and revised. Procedures need to be implemented, and rules must be enforced. Many institutions are already struggling to adequately oversee their research, and many individuals already feel that the administrative burden of research is too high. Conflict-of-interest management can further stretch already limited resources and energy. Yet, if the threats to research quality and trust posed by financial interests are taken seriously, then institutions and individuals need to recognize that these tangible and intangible costs necessarily accompany the otherwise beneficial relationships and activities that generate financial conflicts of interest in the first place.

If current management systems are streamlined, simplified, and better enforced, they will become more effective. They may also receive better support from those they regulate (as well as from those concerned to critique the prevalence of financial interests in biomedical research). Without improved support for the policies, improved management will be extremely difficult, apart from cost concerns.

The types of management system currently employed in biomedical research cannot function without a level of general support from all involved. Because these systems rely on self-reporting and, to a great degree, self- and peer regulation, they will not work unless those involved understand and accept the rationale for those systems. As law professor Robert Gatter (2003, 389) noted, "Law and norms literature recognizes that the more conduct is controlled by rules imposed outside of a community of actors, the more actors inside that community will act out of self-interest and without regard to the normative basis of those rules."

There is some worrisome evidence that support for current management is mixed. When the NIH instituted its strict consulting rules, some employees expressed significant opposition. A survey of almost 2,000 faculty members at the (then) nine University of California campuses revealed limited understanding of important details of policies and some lack of support for these policies (Lipton, Boyd, and Bero 2004). The survey found strong distrust of the process among "a vocal minority" and "a belief in the ability of individuals to recognize and, if necessary, reduce their own conflicts of interest, without the intervention of the institution" (98). Conflict-of-interest management cannot succeed if biomedical researchers confuse conflicts of interest with bias, do not believe that conflicts of interest pose threats to biomedical research's quality and trustworthiness, believe they can manage those threats without policies or rules, or believe there should be no limits on the kinds of financial interest they can hold. Sometimes, avoiding a conflict of interest will mean forgoing personal or institutional financial gain, which must be accepted for the necessary cultural change to succeed.

If similar levels of misunderstanding and negative feeling are widespread in the research community, improvements in the knowledge and understanding of and support for financial conflict-of-interest management will require: (1) simplifying, improving, and better enforcing policies; (2) improving communication of and education about those policies; and (3) otherwise promoting acceptance within the culture of biomedical research through education, continuing education, and internal leadership. Insofar as there is a lack of "buy-in" within the biomedical research community regarding the importance of avoiding or otherwise managing conflicts of interest, education can help explain why conflicts of interest are considered problematic and describe the risks posed to research quality and, particularly, to public trust by a failure to respond. Education should draw on the existing data, but it will also need to thoroughly explain why the threat to trust, on which there are currently few data, is considered so important. Researchers steeped in a data- and evidence-based world may easily understand the threat to research quality of investigator judgment consciously or unconsciously influenced by financial concerns. They may be less easily convinced that research seeming to lack objectivity represents a profound threat to trust and that trust is an essential element of the biomedical research system.

To the extent that a norm against financial conflicts of interest already exists in the biomedical research community, it has much in common with Merton's norms of disinterestedness and communalism, valuing both actual and apparent impartiality and disvaluing impediments to open communication and sharing of knowledge. Education alone cannot create (or strengthen) this norm. The norm can be strengthened and maintained only by the community, a task that is made more difficult by the overall context within which biomedical research takes place—a context that encourages researchers and institutions to pursue a range of research funding and to capture intellectual property rights as often as possible.

Nevertheless, something may be learned from professions that censure those who hide or fail to address their financial (and other) conflicts of interest (Davis and Johnston 2009). Aside from a number of clearly prohibited situations, these professions do not usually condemn individuals or institutions for being in a financial conflict of interest per se, but censure instead the inappropriate or inadequate management of that situation. Such a culture uses written rules to communicate a preexisting internal norm, which is then enforced through individual conscience and the risk of peer disapproval and, in some cases, through legal action or professional sanction (e.g., disbarment or formal reprimand). The rules would not work without widespread acceptance and support from the community.

No one likes to be told that he or she cannot be trusted to resist the sway of money, and yet lawyers, judges, accountants, engineers, architects, journalists, and other professionals long ago acknowledged the need to avoid or manage financial conflicts of interest. For many of these professionals, a culture of embarrassment backs clearly articulated norms and sometimes very detailed rules requiring the complete avoidance of certain conflicts of interest and the disclosure and further management of others. Accepting that certain financial arrangements must be avoided, divested, disclosed, or otherwise managed need not be an admission of weakness, deviance, or sloppy morals. Instead, it can be the hallmark of a commitment to rigorously maintaining integrity and remaining above reproach.

ACKNOWLEDGMENT

This research was funded by the Patrick and Catherine Weldon Donaghue Medical Research Foundation.

REFERENCES

AAMC Task Force on Financial Conflicts of Interest in Clinical Research. 2001. *Protecting Subjects, Preserving Trust, Promoting Progress: Policy and Guidelines for the Oversight of Individual Financial Interests in Human Subjects Research.* Washington, DC: Association of American Medical Colleges.

———. 2002. *Protecting Subjects, Preserving Trust, Promoting Progress II: Principles and Recommendations for Oversight of an Institution's Financial Interests in Human Subjects Research.* Washington, DC: Association of American Medical Colleges.

American Society of Clinical Oncology. 2003. Revised conflict of interest policy. *Journal of Clinical Oncology* 21 (12): 1–3.

American Society of Gene Therapy. 2000. *Policy of the American Society of Gene Therapy on Financial Conflict of Interest in Clinical Research.* Milwaukee, WI: American Society of Gene Therapy.

Ancker, J. S., and A. Flanagin. 2007. A comparison of conflict of interest policies at peer reviewed journals in different scientific disciplines. *Science and Engineering Ethics* 13 (2): 147–57.

Angell, M. 2000. Is academic medicine for sale? *New England Journal of Medicine* 342 (20): 1516–18.

Association of American Universities. 2001. *Report on Individual and Institutional Financial Conflict of Interest.* Washington, DC: Association of American Universities.

Bekelman, J. E., Y. Li, and C. P. Gross. 2003. Scope and impact of financial conflicts of interest in biomedical research: A systematic review. *JAMA* 289 (4): 454–65.

Bero, L. A., and D. Rennie. 1996. Influences on the quality of published drug studies. *International Journal of Technological Assessment in Health Care* 12 (2): 209–37.

Blumenthal, D., E. G. Campbell, M. S. Anderson, N. Causino, and K. S. Louis. 1997. Withholding research results in academic life science: Evidence from a national survey of faculty. *JAMA* 277 (15): 1224–28.

Blumenthal, D., N. Causino, E. Campbell, and K. S. Louis. 1996. Relationships between academic institutions and industry in the life sciences: An industry survey. *New England Journal of Medicine* 334 (6): 368–73.

Bok, D. 2003. *Universities in the Marketplace: The Commercialization of Higher Education.* Princeton, NJ: Princeton University Press.

Brody, B. A., C. Anderson, S. V. McCrary, L. McCullough, R. Morgan, and N. Wray. 2003. Expanding disclosure of conflicts of interest: The views of stakeholders. *IRB* 25 (1): 1–8.

Campbell, E. G., B. R. Clarridge, M. Gokhale, L. Birenbaum, S. Hilgartner, N. A. Holtzman, and D. Blumenthal. 2002. Data withholding in academic genetics: Evidence from a national survey. *JAMA* 287 (4): 473–80.

Campbell, E. G., G. Koski, and D. Blumenthal. 2004. *The Triple Helix: University, Government, and Industry Relationships in the Life Sciences.* Washington, DC: AEI-Brookings Joint Center for Regulatory Studies.

Campbell, E., G. Koski, D. E. Zinner, and D. Blumenthal. 2005. Managing the triple helix in the life sciences. *Issues in Science and Technology,* Winter: 48–54.

Campbell, E. G., J. S. Weissman, S. Ehringhaus, S. R. Rao, B. Moy, S. Feibelmann, and S. Dorr Goold. 2007. Institutional academic-industry relationships. *JAMA* 298 (15): 1779–86.

Chaudhry, S., S. Schroter, R. Smith, and J. Morris. 2002. Does declaration of competing interests affect readers' perceptions? A randomised trial. *BMJ* 325 (7377): 1391–92.

Cho, M. K., R. Shohara, A. Schissel, and D. Rennie. 2000. Policies on faculty conflicts of interest at US universities. *JAMA* 284 (17): 2203–8.

Cooper, R. J., M. Gupta, M. S. Wilkes, and J. R. Hoffman. 2006. Conflict of interest disclosure policies and practices in peer-reviewed biomedical journals. *Journal of General Internal Medicine* 21 (12): 1248–52.

Davidson, R. A. 1986. Source of funding and outcome of clinical trials. *Journal of General Internal Medicine* 1 (3): 155–58.

Davis, M., and J. Johnston. 2009. Appendix C: Conflict of interest in four professions: A comparative analysis. In *Conflict of Interest in Medical Research, Education, and Practice,* ed. B. Lo and M. J. Field. Washington, DC: Institute of Medicine, National Academies Press.

Davis, M., and A. Stark. 2001. *Conflict of Interest in the Professions.* New York: Oxford University Press.

Drazen, J. M., and G. D. Curfman. 2002. Financial associations of authors. *New England Journal of Medicine* 346 (24): 1901–2.

Etzkowitz, H. 2002. *MIT and the Rise of Entrepreneurial Science.* New York: Routledge.

Federation of American Societies for Experimental Biology. 2006. *Shared Responsibility, Individual Integrity: Scientists Addressing Conflicts of Interest in Biomedical Research.* Mar. 13. Washington, DC: Federation of American Societies for Experimental Biology.

Friedberg, M., B. Saffran, T. J. Stinson, W. Nelson, and C. L. Bennett. 1999. Evaluation of conflict of interest in economic analyses of new drugs used in oncology. *JAMA* 282 (15): 1453–57.

Gatter, R. 2003. Walking the talk of trust in human subjects research: The challenge of regulating financial conflicts of interest. *Emory Law Journal* 52 (1): 327–401.

Glynn, M. L. 2004. Letter to the co-chairman of a panel, dated Apr. 19, 2004. Office of Government Ethics. www.usoge.gov

Hamermesh, D. 2002. The annual report on the economic status of the profession 2001–02. *Academe* 88 (2): 20–42.

Hardin, R. 2002. *Trust and Trustworthiness.* New York: Russell Sage Foundation.

Harris, G., and A. Berenson. 2005. 10 voters on panel backing pain pills had industry ties. *New York Times*, Feb. 25.

Harris, G., and B. Carey. 2008. Researchers fail to reveal full drug pay. *New York Times*, June 8.

Institute of Medicine. 2009. *Conflict of Interest in Medical Research, Education, and Practice.* Washington, DC: National Academies Press.

Johnston, J. 2004. Outing the conflicted: *et tu,* NIH? *Science* 303 (5664): 1610.

Kennedy, D. 2006. Good news—and bad. *Science* 311 (5758): 145.

Kjaergard, L. L., and B. Als-Nielsen. 2002. Association between competing interests and authors' conclusions: Epidemiological study of randomised clinical trials published in the BMJ. *BMJ* 325 (7358): 249.

Knight, J. 2003. Accusations of bias prompt NIH review of ethical guidelines. *Nature* 426 (6968): 741.

Krimsky, S. 2003. *Science in the Private Interest: Has the Lure of Profits Corrupted Biomedical Research?* Lanham, MD: Rowman & Littlefield.

Krimsky, S., and L. S. Rothenberg. 2001. Conflict of interest policies in science and medical journals: Editorial practices and author disclosures. *Science and Engineering Ethics* 7 (2): 205–18.

Lipton, S., E. A. Boyd, and L. A. Bero. 2004. Conflicts of interest in academic research: Policies, processes, and attitudes. *Accountability in Research* 11 (2): 83–102.

Medical Economics Company. 1995. *Physicians' Desk Reference Medical Dictionary.* 1st ed. Montvale, NJ: Medical Economics.

Merton, R. K. 1973 [1942]. The normative structure of science. In *The Sociology of Science: Theoretical and Empirical Investigations,* ed. R. K. Merton, 267–80. Chicago: University of Chicago Press.

Moses, H., III, E. R. Dorsey, D. H. Matheson, S. O. Thier, and J. B. Martin. 2005. Financial anatomy of biomedical research. *JAMA* 295 (9): 999–1000.

Moses, H., III, and J. B. Martin. 2001. Academic relationships with industry: A new model for biomedical research. *JAMA* 285 (7): 933–35.

National Institutes of Health and Office of Extramural Research. 2002. Financial conflict of interest: Objectivity in research. http://grants.nih.gov.

National Science Board. 2008. *Science and Engineering Indicators.* 2 vols (vol. 1, NSB 08-1; vol. 2, NSB 08-1A). Arlington, VA: National Science Foundation.

Nelson, D., and R. Weiss. 2000. Penn researchers sued in gene therapy death. *Washington Post,* Sept. 19.

Office of Technology Transfer and National Institutes of Health. 2008. Statistics. http://ott.od .nih.gov/index.aspx.

Press, E., and. J. Washburn. 2000. The kept university. *Atlantic Monthly,* Mar.: 39.

Rochon, P. A., J. H. Gurwitz, C. M. Cheung, J. A. Hayes, and T. C. Chalmers. 1994. Evaluating the quality of articles published in journal supplements compared with the quality of those published in the parent journal. *JAMA* 272 (2): 108–13.

Rosenberg, N., and R. Nelson. 1994. American research universities and technical advance in industry. *Research Policy* 23 (3): 323–48.

Sage, W. M. 2007. Some principles require principals: Why banning "conflicts of interest" won't solve incentive problems in biomedical research. *Texas Law Review* 85 (6): 1413–63.

Steinbrook, R. 2004. Financial conflicts of interest and the NIH. *New England Journal of Medicine* 350 (4): 327–30.

Stelfox, H. T., G. Chua, K. O'Rourke, and A. S. Detsky. 1998. Conflict of interest in the debate of calcium-channel antagonists. *New England Journal of Medicine* 338 (2):101.

Stevens, A. J., and F. Toneguzzo, eds. 2004. *AUTM Licensing Survey, FY 2003: Survey Summary.* Deerfield, IL: Association of University Technology Managers.

Stevens, A. J., F. Toneguzzo, and D. Bostrom, eds. 2005. *AUTM U.S. Licensing Survey, FY 2004: Survey Summary.* Deerfield, IL: Association of University Technology Managers.

Stossel, T. P. 2005. Regulating academic-industrial research relationships: Solving problems or stifling progress? *New England Journal of Medicine* 353 (10): 1060–65.

Tanner, L. 2006. JAMA says it was misled by researchers. Associated Press. July 12.

Thompson, D. F. 1993. Understanding financial conflicts of interest. *New England Journal of Medicine* 329 (8): 573–76.

Thornton, S. 2009. On the brink: The annual report on the economic status of the profession, 2008–09. *Academe* 95 (2): 14–28.

Tieckelmann, R., R. Kordal, and D. Bostrom, eds. 2008. *AUTM U.S. Licensing Activity Survey, FY2007: A Survey Summary of Technology Licensing (and Related) Activity for U.S. Academic and Nonprofit Institutions and Technology Investment Firms.* Deerfield, IL: Association of University Technology Managers.

U.S. Department of Health and Human Services. 2001. *Draft Interim Guidance "Financial Relationships and Interests in Research Involving Human Subjects: Guidance for Human Subject Protection."* Washington, DC: U.S. Department of Health and Human Services. www.hhs.gov.

———. 2004. Financial relationships and interests in research involving human subjects: Guidance for human subject protection. *Federal Register* 69 (92): 26393–97.

U.S. Federal Housing Finance Agency. 2009. *House Price Index.* Washington, DC: Federal Housing Finance Agency. www.fhfa.gov.

U.S. Food and Drug Administration. 1998. 21 CFR Part 54: Financial disclosure by clinical investigators. *Federal Register* 63 (Feb. 2): 5250–54.

U.S. General Accounting Office. 2001. *HHS Direction Needed to Address Financial Conflicts of Interest.* Washington, DC: U.S. General Accounting Office.

U.S. Office of Government Ethics. 2004. *Review of the Ethics Program at the National Institutes of Health.* Washington, DC: U.S. Office of Government Ethics.

U.S. Public Health Service. 1996. 42 CFR Part 50, Subpart F: Responsibility of applicants for promoting objectivity in research for which PHS funding is sought. *Federal Register* 61: 174–76.

Washburn, J. 2005. *University, Inc.: The Corporate Corruption of American Higher Education.* New York: Basic Books.

Willman, D. 2003a. Records of payments to NIH staff sought. *Los Angeles Times*, Dec. 9.

———. 2003b. Stealth merger: Drug companies and government medical research. *Los Angeles Times*, Dec. 7.

World Medical Association. 2008. *World Medical Association Declaration of Helsinki—Ethical Principles for Medical Research Involving Human Subjects.* 6th rev. Ferney-Voltaire, France: World Medical Association. www.wma.net.

CHAPTER 2

Conflicts between Commercial and Scientific Roles in Academic Health Research

NEETIKA PRABHAKAR COX, M.P.P.,
CHRISTOPHER HEANEY, B.A.,
AND ROBERT M. COOK-DEEGAN, M.D.

Gov'r. Thomas was so pleas'd with the construction of this stove . . . that he offered to give me a patent for the sole vending of them for a term of years; but I declin'd it from a principle which has ever weighed with me on such occasions, viz., That, as we enjoy great advantages from the inventions of others, we should be glad of an opportunity to serve others by any invention of ours; and this we should do freely and generously.

—*The Autobiography of Benjamin Franklin*, pt. XVII

In April 2003, John Sulston—as the U.K. scientist most strongly associated with the just-completed reference sequence of the human genome—commemorated the fiftieth anniversary of the discovery of the double-helical structure of DNA by giving a lecture to a throng of Nobel laureates and others. He stood on his home turf at the epicenter of global molecular biology, the University of Cambridge, just blocks from where Watson and Crick did their work (and even closer to the Eagle Pub, where Crick announced discovering "the secret of life"). Sulston extolled the virtues of making the reference sequence available to all, at no charge, and pointed to the myriad ways in which sequence data would be translated into human benefit, not just in the form of new knowledge, but also as goods, services, jobs, and wealth. He made a case for the practical commercial value and economic efficiency of having a robust public domain, based mainly on the arguments that network economies are powerful means for sharing fundamental scientific data.

Weeks later, James Davis, of Human Genome Sciences, Inc. (HGS), addressed patent aficionados assembled around a table at Resources for the Future, in Washington, DC, at a meeting convened by the American Association for the Advancement of Science (Davis 2003). He told of the immense value of patents as a stimulus for biomedical innovation, citing the example of a gene for which his company was seeking patent protection directly linked to three products for treating cardiovascular disease. He noted that the prospect of a patent—with its power to exclude others from making, using, selling, or importing products based on the gene—induced investment in his company and that, without strong patent protection, the company would be hard put to pay for the extensive clinical trials and product testing needed to get Food and Drug Administration approval.

Both Sulston and Davis are right. And both are wrong, if they believe theirs are the only paths to innovation. If either set of rules were generalized to all health research, the system of innovation would be diminished. Davis's rules would constrict the public domain to small pastures surrounded by high fences enclosing intellectual property. Sulston's rules would restrict innovation to public works. (To be fair, both men give a nod to select cases where the alternative framework makes sense—Sulston to the commercial value of gene patents for some end products, and Davis to the value of open academic research—but their policy prescriptions belie the nodding.)

A powerful but complex system of public and privately funded health research has developed over the past two decades. A large and consistent infusion of public dollars for decades after World War II gave way, by the early 1990s, to rough parity between government and private support for health research and development (R&D), with most of the private health R&D in pharmaceuticals, biotechnology, and medical devices. The government funds health research to improve health; private R&D funding has ridden a wave of increased spending on drugs, devices, and biologics in the health sector and lucrative markets for those products. The result is more science, more goods and services, a larger fraction of the economy devoted to health and health research—and ample opportunity for conflicts of interest.

Academic research institutions are where public and private health R&D meet. Academic research promotes health outcomes by producing knowledge through research, which in turn feeds into development in private firms. Academic research centers are valuable because the knowledge they produce is tied to the training of future health professionals, future scientists, and future industry researchers and managers. The academic sector is the main performer of publicly funded research. Its health is vital to the private sector, which depends heavily on open science—and can even take it for granted.

The complexities of public and private involvement in health research are reflected in the differences between Davis's and Sulston's visions of openness, secrecy, and patenting. The benefits of the open-disclosure rules governing the public Human Genome Project, as espoused by Sulston, are real. But universally mandated open disclosure for all research would make creation of companies such as HGS impossible, because no one would invest in their creation. If, on the other hand, the Human Genome Project had progressed in the same style as HGS, little sequence information would be publicly available; that kind of project would have been close to useless except to the owner of the data.

HGS has disclosed only a miniscule fraction of its decade's worth of DNA sequence and other data. Who would expect it to do more? But is that how we want science in general to progress? Of course not. Scientific progress building on only HGS sequence data would slow to a crawl, because so few could use the information. If private funding were the only source of support for sequencing data, every company would retain the data behind walls of secrecy until they became public through an issued patent or publication of a patent application—or until the company decided to make the data available to establish scientific credentials or for some other reason. Scientists who were not working at companies that purchased access to the data would have only their own data to examine. A system of privately held data would be incredibly expensive, wasteful, and slow by comparison with Sulston's "science commons," available to all. The conflicts that erupt over access to data are intensifying precisely because data are valuable, both for public health and for private fortune.

Academic scientists often stand at a point where the norms of open science confront a strong pull to keep data proprietary. At this point, the role of academic scientists committed to openness conflicts with a commercial role as a link in a private R&D chain.

Patents figure in the value of discovery and also in role conflicts. If HGS had no prospect of patents, it and hundreds of companies whose business plans are premised on patenting DNA-based inventions might not exist. The products and services they develop would be much longer in coming, as would the social benefits those goods and services confer.

The real world has both open and proprietary science operating in parallel, applied to different projects funded by different entities to accomplish different purposes. *Vive la différence.* But the fact that current policies permit both public, open research and private, proprietary research does not imply that such policies are optimal—or that we have thought carefully about how to attain maximal social benefit. Indeed, it is hard to argue that the current system is anywhere near its peak efficiency, with drug-discovery productivity (measured in products per dollar) plummeting, expenditures rising (Pharmaceutical Research and Manufacturers of America 2009), and the scientific community increasingly complaining about strictures on sharing of data and materials (Lei, Juneja, and Wright 2009). Genomics R&D is being pulled in many different directions at once, some forces pulling toward openness, some toward secrecy. And that is just genomics, which is merely a case study for a general problem confronting health R&D and, for that matter, R&D in general.

In this chapter we review the context in which biomedical research is conducted, highlighting those features that intensify conflicts between norms of Mertonian open science (Merton 1973 [1942]) and commercial, private research and development. We review some facts and figures about health research in the period since World War II and then turn to observations about the context in which issues of "conflict of interest" have been framed.

The conflicting roles of academic scientists may or may not be best framed as "conflicts of interest," with interests strictly defined as fiduciary duties of professionals to their clients, but they exemplify real conflicts among the contending goals of academic health research. Conflicts arise because the people involved wear many hats. A single biomedical research academic might serve as principal investigator, industrial consultant, policy advisor, advisor to venture and angel investors, advisor (or even officer) in funding new ventures, corporate officer, and grant reviewer. As science moves forward and becomes more complex, so too do the issues of policy and entrepreneurship that surround it.

Conflicts between academic and commercial norms, and, more specifically, tensions between sharing data and materials or keeping them secret, arise in at least three ways. First, secrecy within academic research conflicts with norms of openness. Those norms serve an important social purpose, because the "science commons" on which all science grazes—both public and private—depends on publication to make data available for verification and cumulative advance. The training of students is also much stronger, and standard-setting for common technologies much easier, when information is in the open and not hidden behind walls of secrecy. Second, the self-interest of scientists and scientific institutions may provide incentives to act for personal gain, which can conflict with the trust placed in academic science to be a pillar of truth in a neutral, objective system aiming to maximize social benefit. When academic clinicians write review articles that discuss which drugs work for whom, they are acting as judges. But in academic health research under current rules, the judges may be "on the take," in the damning words of former *New England Journal of Medicine* editor Jerome Kassirer (2004). Third, the systems for deciding research priorities and overseeing the research process can introduce biases that promote industrial interests over academic values. If researchers are pursuing a hidden commercial agenda in helping plan the expenditure of public resources or in selecting projects through peer review—by promoting their own interests or throwing spokes in competitors' wheels—they threaten the system's integrity. In this role as sculptors that shape R&D, scientists' commercial interests merely intensify long-standing conflicts in research, based on scientific priority and academic prestige, but in a way that the general public is especially apt to recognize as corrupting. Money is easy to understand, while scientific and academic reputation is more abstruse.

Conflicts for institutions, as well as for individual scientists and clinicians, can arise between their roles as industrial partners and as neutral, objective arbiters of truth (Association of American Medical Colleges 2001, 2002). Where institutional roles conflict, conflicts for academic researchers are sure to follow. Health researchers, like all human beings, respond to institutional incentives, sometimes with exquisite sensitivity.

More Money in Research

Since World War II, federal appropriations for R&D have increased spectacularly. National Institutes of Health (NIH) appropriations alone have grown from less than $1 million in 1942 to more than $35 billion in 2009 (figure 2.1). Before the war, the conventional wisdom in academic medicine was that the government did not have an appropriate place in the world of science and that government funding would mean government control (Smith 1990). As

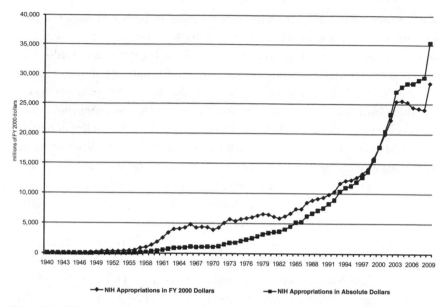

Figure 2.1. NIH appropriations, 1940–2009. *Note:* The 2009 figure includes $5 billion, or half the "stimulus" funding for NIH, available for FY 2009 and FY 2010. Figures are shown in both absolute dollars and adjusted by the Office of Management and Budget's deflator to constant FY 2000 dollars. *Sources:* Data through 2007 based on appropriations reported by the NIH (2009a); data for 2008 and 2009 based on the president's 2010 budget request as reported by the NIH (2009b).

science's practical value became increasingly apparent during the war, reliance on industry for development and production and on universities for research was established (National Research Council 1995). Bruce Smith (1990, 37) noted that "the incentives of the marketplace would continue to spur innovative activity, and the manufacturing strength of U.S. industry would ensure high-quality products and quick exploitation of market opportunities." Industry had always been involved, but after the war, the practical benefit of federal funding for academic research became a founding principle of science policy. A closer relationship between science, government, and industry emerged, as attention shifted from winning a war to sustaining U.S. economic growth (Mowery et al. 2004).

The growing thirst for innovation required investment on a grand scale. The costs were too great to be borne by philanthropy alone. Government became the bulwark support for scientific research, with universities playing a large role as research institutions, especially in areas with clear federal missions such as national defense and public health. In the decades following the war, the federal government became the dominant sponsor of health research (Institute of Medicine 1990).

The increase in R&D after World War II spawned commercialization, first in hard-technology industries and later in enterprises concerned with chemicals, pharmaceuticals, biomedical devices, and biotechnology. The rise in privately funded health research gained momentum in the 1980s. The links between technological innovation and economic opportunity became apparent; the marriage between industrial innovation and academic research was consummated, and this relationship entailed increasingly frequent intercourse.

Eventually, however, the increasing connections also raised questions about economic opportunism at the expense of the academic mission of universities, hospitals, and nonprofit research centers, which were increasingly tightly linked to corporate interests. Onlookers became concerned about what was happening behind closed doors.

Shifts in the Culture of Funding

The net social value of academic health research as a whole is not controversial. Growth in funding for health research in the United States has consistently prevailed under both political parties for six decades, reflecting a strong, shared belief in its social and economic value. Academic health research has a long and storied history, but it was pursued on a relatively small scale until the middle of the twentieth century.

Before World War II, most health research was funded by industry (55%), particularly the pharmaceutical industry (figure 2.2). Most "public" funding for basic biology and health research came from private philanthropies (38%), and government was a bit player (7%) (Ginzburg and Dutka 1989; Dustira 1992). By the mid-1960s, the federal government had become the dominant funder (68%), displacing private industry (24%) and philanthropy (8%). Then, by the start of the twenty-first century, industry (48%) was once again larger than government (44%), and private philanthropy, while it had grown in absolute terms, was a smaller fraction (8%) (Global Forum for Health Research 2001, 2008; Cook-Deegan and McGeary 2006). The NIH budget, which was $464,000 in 1939, surged into the billions during the 1970s and exceeded $35 billion by 2009 (National Institutes of Health 2009b). Private health R&D grew slowly until the 1980s, and there was no significant bio-

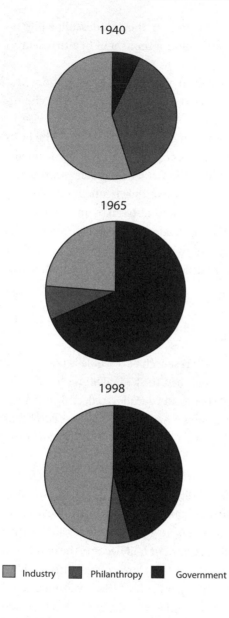

1940

1965

1998

Industry   Philanthropy   Government

Figure 2.2. Industry, philanthropy, and government funding of health research, 1940, 1965, and 1998. *Sources:* Data for 1940 from Dustira 1992; data for 1965 from Ginzburg and Dutka 1989; data for 1998 from Global Forum for Health Research 2001.

technology industry until the early 1980s. For three decades, from the 1950s into the 1980s, the federal government basically ran the show. Corporate science did not change fundamentally in its norms and practices; it was always private and kept chugging along, but public science grew by leaps and bounds.

A generation of health researchers, now in their late career phase, built their careers on expectations of continuing growth. Many of them gained prominence during the period of federal dominance in the mid-1970s, when the norms of science were public values close to the "universal" and "communal" norms that Merton extolled.

In the period leading up to and following World War II, a series of fateful policy decisions were made in government, among private health research advocates, and in academic research centers. These decisions shaped six decades of expansion in health research (see figure 2.1).

Policies in the United States are of particular interest, for four reasons. First, the level of investment in health research is larger in the United States than in any other country. In Global Forum for Health Research surveys (2008), the United States accounts for half of the world's total of government and nonprofit health research funding. Second, expenditures on health goods and services are larger in the United States than any other country, both in absolute terms and as a fraction of gross domestic product (GDP) and per capita GDP (Organization for Economic Cooperation and Development 2008). Thus the U.S. market for drugs, devices, procedures, and other health goods and services is the largest on the planet and is, in that sense, the main driver of biomedical innovation. The lack of direct government price controls for health goods and services is also an important factor, making profits higher in the United States than elsewhere—although other governments vary widely in how directly they set prices, so this is not a consistent difference. Third, the United States has a distinctive framework for academic-industrial mutualism, a major theme of this chapter. This framework includes the Bayh-Dole Act and other formal federal statutory law (Mowery et al. 2004), as well as the regulations and norms that embody "technology transfer" in the United States. The growth of formal "technology transfer" historically parallels the growth of biotechnology and the rapid growth of industry's health research investment in the 1980s. Molecular biology may have been Mertonian at birth, but it was brought up under capitalism.

The fourth reason that health R&D in the United States is particularly significant is that most health research and development takes place there—not just the funding, but the R&D itself. The United States is home to the institutions that do most of the world's health research. This is true in academia, but is also true *a fortiori* for private health R&D, even for companies with headquarters outside the United States.

Dependence of Private Health R&D on Academic Research

The scientific orientation of the pharmaceutical industry is a worldwide phenomenon, but it is most concentrated in the United States and Europe. The rise of private pharmaceutical R&D in the United States accelerated in the early 1980s, exceeding public funding for health research by the end of that decade, according to pharmaceutical industry figures (figure 2.3).

In addition to this scientific turn taken by pharmaceutical R&D in the 1980s, publicly funded science gave rise to a new technological sector—biotechnology—starting in the United States, Japan, and Europe and spreading globally, but developing most exuberantly in the United States (U.S. Congress, Office of Technology Assessment 1984, 1991). Academic research in molecular and cellular biology of the 1960s and 1970s spawned the new biotechnology in the early 1980s, and industrial biotechnology still has its largest presence in the United States.

Academic-Industrial Mutualism

The economic sectors and industries most relevant to human health are unusually dependent on publicly funded science performed at academic research institutions. One way to document this dependency is to trace the history of major innovations. The classic TRACES study, funded by the National Science Foundation (NSF), for example, looked at several important discoveries. These included a few related to human health, such as development of the birth control pill and of the electron microscope so widely used in biomedical research (Illinois Institute of Technology Research Institute 1968). One large and elaborate study of the same era, the Comroe-Dripps study, emphasized the importance of academic research in ten major advances in treating heart disease (Comroe and Dripps 1976, 1977). Many stories in the National Academy of Sciences' *Beyond Discovery* series (2003) are about health research, showing how practical application drew on academic science. The Association of University Technology Managers (AUTM) has collected narratives about university inventions in reports in its "Better World Project" (2006–9). Health research is a major source of such stories. The studies and reports fall short of producing a highly predictive model of biomedical innovation or an input-output matrix that can be specified in detail. Nonetheless, they amply demonstrate the value of academic research in developing new

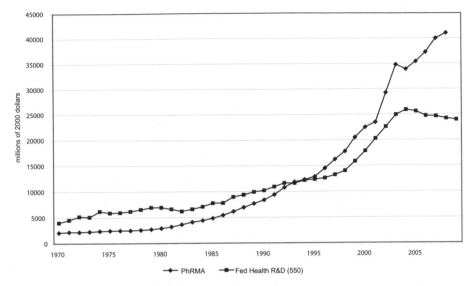

Figure 2.3. Federal health R&D (budget function 550) versus pharmaceutical industry R&D (according to PhRMA, Pharmaceutical Research and Manufacturers of America), 1970–2008. *Sources:* Data on federal budget function 550 for 1970–2008 from the National Science Foundation (1999, 2001a, 2001b, 2002, 2004a, 2004b, 2006a, 2006b, 2007, 2008) and president's budget request for FY 2009 as reported by the NIH (2009b); data on PhRMA R&D expenditures from annual surveys (Pharmaceutical Research and Manufacturers of America 2009; past surveys on file with authors), deflated according to the Office of Management and Budget's GDP deflator from the president's budget request for FY 2010, historical table 10.1 (Office of Management and Budget 2009).

products and services to improve medical care. Case studies instantiate the conventional wisdom that academic health research has practical value.

Empirical studies of innovation also point to the immense value of "open science" for private commerce, particularly in pharmaceuticals and biotechnology. Economist Edwin Mansfield (1995) queried industrial executives about the degree to which their products relied wholly or partly on academic science. The responses from pharmaceutical executives stood out: in this sector, twice as many products either would not have been developed or would have been substantially delayed without academic research, compared with other industrial sectors. The survey results are corroborated by patent data in this unusually patent-dependent sector. Pharmaceutical and biotechnology patents are much more likely to cite academic research than are patents in other sectors (Narin and Rozek 1988; Narin and Olivastro 1992).

Academic institutions not only are cited in more patents but also own more intellectual property in areas related to life sciences, particularly genomics, than in other areas of R&D. In all patent classes as a whole, academic and nonprofit institutions hold fewer than 3 percent of patents, but the proportion climbed to 39 percent for DNA-based patents in the period 1980–93 (S. McCormack, unpublished data). While few in number compared with later academic patents on DNA-based inventions, these early patents include many fundamental genes and methods that proved both widely useful (in both science and industry) and lucrative for the academic institutions that licensed them. The number of academically owned patents has risen steeply in pharmaceuticals, and unlike the drop-off in citations of academic patents in other fields, citation of academic patents in pharmaceutical and medical patent classes has risen over the past two decades (Gambardella 1995; Henderson, Jaffe, and Trajtenberg 1995; Cockburn and Henderson 1996; R. M. Cook-Deegan's subsector analysis of Henderson, Jaffe, and Trajtenberg 1995).[1]

The Roles of Academic Technology Licensing

The 96th Congress passed the Patent and Trademark Law Amendments Act in December 1980, during a lame-duck session (Stevens 2004). This law (Public Law 96-517) is known as the Bayh-Dole Act, for the names of its Senate sponsors, Birch Bayh and Robert Dole. It was passed in reaction to disparate patent-ownership policies among government agencies. Some agencies strongly resisted policies to confer patent rights on federal grantees and contractors (U.S. Department of Health, Education and Welfare 1978). The NIH had developed institutional patent agreements that enabled contractors to retain patent rights, but these agreements were at government discretion and far from universal in health research.

When Cohen and Boyer discovered recombinant DNA, with funding from the NSF and NIH, for example, a vigorous debate ensued about whether their invention should be patented and, if so, whether the patent should be assigned to their universities (Stanford and the University of California) or to the federal government. NIH Director Donald Fredrickson solicited views from universities throughout the country and was deluged with letters, most of them arguing for universities' owning and managing patents resulting from their federally funded work, very much in consonance with the Bayh-Dole framework (Mowery et al. 2004). In the end, the decision was that Stanford and the University of California would prosecute the patents and then own and manage them by licensing to private sector firms (Hughes 2001; Feldman, Colaianni, and Liu 2007). The first of these recombinant DNA patents was granted in the same month that the Bayh-Dole Act passed. The NIH and NSF were already enabling grantees to get patents, moving in the direction of Bayh-Dole, but the Act made the policy more consistent among federal funding agencies and pushed grantee institutions that did not yet have the capacity for technology licensing to develop it (Rosenfeld 1988; Jankowski 1999; Stevens 2004). The new statute directly overrode policies of other agencies, such as the Department of Energy, that favored government ownership of patents arising from federally funded research.

The Bayh-Dole Act actively encouraged academic research institutions to strengthen their ties to industry by giving them clear rights to intellectual property and a mandate to license it. Creating incentives for industrial collaboration was a matter of deliberate policy. The rise in academic patenting is probably due mainly to the increasing relevance of academic science to industry and the increase in federal funding for science, rather than to rules about patent ownership and licensing, but Bayh-Dole certainly simplified the process and lowered transaction costs by setting default ownership rules. If the purpose of Bayh-Dole was to encourage academic institutions to get patents, then the success of this legislation is indisputable, as borne out by patent counts (Rai and Eisenberg 2003; Mowery et al. 2004). If the purpose was to foster innovation, however, the verdict is more nuanced and less decisive (Mowery et al. 2004; So et al. 2009).

Mowery et al. (2004, 1) note that some critical accounts of the Bayh-Dole Act suggest that growth in the patenting and licensing of university inventions has "changed the 'research culture' of U.S. universities, leading to increased secrecy, less sharing of research results, and a shift in the focus of academic research away from fundamental to more applied topics." Normal "open science" such as publications, conferences, and informal communication among researchers is a wider channel for real technology transfer—conveying research inputs to industrial R&D—than is the narrow conception of technology transfer as licensing of patents and other intellectual property. Yet those channels are not as open as they could be, and attention is turning to whether this affects industrial users by constricting information flow. Scientists sometimes deny colleagues' requests for information to protect the patentability or commercial value of their research or because of agreements with industry linked to research support, material transfer or other agreements, or nondisclosure agreements (Campbell et al. 2002; Campbell and Bendavid 2003; Blumenthal et al. 2006; Walsh, Cohen, and Cho 2007; Zinner et al. 2009). To be sure, the main reason not to share is that it is a drain on time and resources, rather than caused by commercial constraints, but commercial incentives add to existing scientific and academic reasons to violate the Mertonian norms.

The Association of University Technology Managers is a professional organization for those who work in the technology transfer (or technology licensing) offices of academic institutions. Its constituency has increased explosively under the Bayh-Dole Act. AUTM's origin stories celebrate the Bayh-Dole statute. Its annual survey data cover the years 1991 through 2008 and are among the few empirical facts available to limn the practices governing academic research outputs relevant to industry. AUTM annual surveys show a dramatic rise in the number of patents and licenses and in the amount of income derived from licenses or cashed-out equity derived from academic research (Association of University Technology Managers 2008). The income from technology licensing per institution varies tremendously. Thursby and Thursby (2007) note that most universities' technology licensing offices barely break even and that many drain rather than contribute to university revenues, but commercialization is a goal of technology licensing, in addition to generation of university revenues. The value of all patents is highly skewed toward a few veins of gold in mountains of less valuable intellectual property. This is as true in academia as elsewhere, and it is partly a matter of luck which universities prosper most. Those with larger research budgets have better odds of hitting a jackpot, but the outcome is unpredictable.

Technology licensing offices serve a multitude of masters. Many contending goals of academic institutions converge on licensing offices, and in the broad sense of potential for conflict among those goals, the licensing offices become the focal point. Some generate institutional revenue, but all are responsible for getting useful results of academic research into the hands of those who can apply them. Licensing income is one measure of success, and indeed, it ranks first among stated goals (Thursby and Thursby 2007), but other goals are also important—most notably, compliance with the commercialization mandate of the Bayh-Dole Act. Efforts to broaden and improve other measures of the impact of the legislation are being developed (Malakoff 2004; Pressman and Walters 2004).

Technology licensing offices are not in a simple game of revenue-maximizing. They are not running a business orthogonal to the university's mission, such as owning a shopping mall or leasing office space. They are, rather, licensing research results produced by the intellectual work of academic faculty and staff. Their work builds directly on the university's research mission. Licensing offices face complex decisions about how to make university-based inventions most valuable. This value includes, but is not restricted to, financial returns to the university. Beyond money, managing patents also includes judgments about scientific and social value. Licensing terms that enable academic research to proceed without royalties are common (Gardner and Garner 2004), and exemptions for use in resource-poor countries are a growing trend.[2] These licensing terms cannot be explained as revenue-maximizing strategies, but rather as strategies intended to promote scientific value (academic use) and social value (use by resource-poor countries). The tools available to licensing offices for making judgments about scientific and social value are imprecise, and solid empirical data about policies are scarce. What is counted—which includes patents, licenses, and revenue streams—is not always what matters most (International Expert Group on Biotechnology, Innovation and Intellectual Property 2008). Recent years have seen more attention to capturing the qualitative aspects of academic discoveries through social impact, usually through documentation of case histories (Lowe and Quick 2004). Empirical research is also increasing (U.S. Department of Health and Human Services, Office of the Inspector General 1995; U.S. General Accounting Office 1999), although empirical measurement remains, and surely will always be, far short of what fully informed decision makers would want.

A scarcity of policy-relevant information is hardly unique to academic-industry ties in the life sciences. Indeed, scarcity of directly pertinent data is the usual case in most policy domains. The fact that money changes hands, patent licenses are counted, and products and services can be quantified does suggest, however, that as technology licensing offices become more computerized, and if AUTM and other groups can set data standards, the base of information for making evidence-based policy choices might grow larger—but that depends on its being open to inspection and sufficiently consistent among institutions to be analyzed.

Good measures of impact are needed to monitor the academic research sector, a key moving part in the engine of innovation. The role of academic research institutions has expanded in the national innovation system, even according to the narrow criterion of supplying useful inventions that get cited and licensed. It is not heartening, therefore, to see the sloppy accounting of government rights to inventions arising from federal funding, as documented in a General Accounting Office report and Inspector General's report in the 1990s (U.S. Department of Health and Human Services, Office of the Inspector General 1994; U.S. General Accounting Office 1999). Both reports show that federal funding agencies do not have the capacity to ensure that the government rights embodied in the Bayh-Dole Act are systematically monitored and enforced. In one case, a surprising fraction of NIH-funded institutions (143 of 633 patents at twelve institutions) had incomplete records with no acknowledgment of a government interest, and in more than half of those "missing acknowledgment" cases, the institutions agreed that government rights should have been acknowledged. A 1994 audit of patents at Scripps Research Institute was even more discouraging (U.S. Department of Health and Human Services, Office of the Inspector General 1994). The inspector general reported that Scripps acknowledged a government interest in only 51 of 125 patents that the inspector general believed involved some federal funding. These data are old, but no new studies have been done, to our knowledge, and independent investigators do not have ready access to the raw data, so it is impossible to know whether the situation has improved.

The Bayh-Dole Act was weak when it came to ensuring that public benefit is foremost in the use of federal dollars. Indeed, the statute is remarkably free of concern for accountability when using public monies. This is true in several respects. There was little attention to transparency of the system, and consequently, the records that government has and that grantees and contractors keep do not supply the feedback that policymakers would need to improve the system over time. Two and a half decades after Bayh-Dole's enactment, few data guide policy, despite our note of optimism above about growing attention to measuring the impacts of technology transfer. AUTM commendably initiated its own effort to gather information about patent counts and licensing revenues, which are surely relevant to both the institutions and the government. Those making policy decisions are even more interested, however, in numbers and types of jobs created, in how much the effective commercial translation of a research tool saved (or cost) the national research system, in how many lives were saved by a new drug, or in how research inputs boosted productivity and economic growth. Moreover, policymakers should want to know not just what happens with licensed technologies, but also what the research institutions do with the revenues generated, given that the statute stipulates they should go toward the public purposes of education and research. Education and research are what academic research institutions do, but they also do many other things, and documenting what happens with revenues would probably produce evidence that reinforces the story that licensing revenue begets more research of social value.

Documenting what universities do with the monies generated from technology licensing could become an innovative form of accountability that does not amount to bean-counting, but traces how the money derived from technology licensing gets channeled into research and education to make a difference. If such uses comport with academic norms, including the support of open science and the pursuit of public benefit, monitoring would acknowledge those uses and encourage more of them.

Calls for accountability and transparency are subject to an important caveat. Broad social impacts are difficult to measure. And even if they can be measured, there is a natural tendency to attribute all the value to only one input—the one being studied, such as the federally funded research that may indeed be innovation's farthest upstream tributary, or the act of licensing a particular technology, which occurs a bit farther downstream. Analysis that gives short shrift to the hundreds of other, less exalted inputs that flow into successful innovation will produce misleading policy implications.

Licensing practices, until recently, have been mainly subject to norms of a relatively narrow technology licensing community. That is now changing, as advocates and activists, nongovernment watchdogs, and investigative reporters are beginning to turn their attention to academic technology transfer policy. It is well past time to open up the system so that we can better learn how it works, with an eye to improving it. The insiders have good ideas about how to do this, but they also have vested interests and can benefit from some sunshine. Attention will be welcomed by enlightened technology licensing officers, but the policies that can ensure transparency and accountability are not yet in place.

Individual Conflict of Interest for Faculty and Staff

If technology licensing offices are the places where most role conflicts converge for academic institutions, individual conflict of interest is a separate but related issue for faculty and staff. The link is institutional oversight of those individuals.

Individual conflict of interest is most often conceived as a problem to be addressed by disclosure policies, with individual faculty reporting to institutional administrators, who may in turn call on "conflict-of-interest committees" for policy advice, as a review mechanism, or both. Conditions of employment as faculty or staff at research institutions may stipulate some practices that are "out of bounds," or they may review proposed arrangements between employees and outside firms case by case, subject to general guidelines. Faculty and staff manuals at most research institutions give at least general guidance, and some define specific prohibited practices. To date, research institutions have mainly relied on their faculty and staff to report proposed relationships as the trigger for such oversight. An analysis of practices at campuses of the University of California found similar procedures but considerable variation in standards and interpretation (Boyd, Lipton, and Bero 2004). A survey of investigators found disgruntlement, sometimes quite passionate, with how conflict-of-interest reporting and review procedures were implemented (Goozner 2004).

Disclosure faces at least two problems: incompleteness and insufficiency. First, disclosure, even public disclosure, may not protect against bias as is intended—its effect may be insufficient or even perverse. Publication of relationships between authors and firms whose products and services are reviewed is now required by many journals. A report of the Center for Science in the Public Interest found that many authors were not reporting financial ties that could be discovered through publicly available information, indicating that such reporting is incomplete—and apt to be incomplete in circumstances where it might be problematic (Cain, Lowenstein, and Moore 2005).

Empirical studies of conflict-of-interest disclosure began to appear in 2006 as part of the Conflict of Interest Notification Study. The studies include surveys of institutional officials and of those who might participate in research. Institutions varied in their disclosure policies and in the degree to which written policies were clear and specific; those with the most specific written policies had the smallest gaps between institutional policy guidance and actual practice as gleaned from interviews (Weinfurt et al. 2006). The Association of American Medical Colleges (AAMC) has been particularly engaged in addressing conflicts of interest, through its guidelines for individual and institutional conflicts of interest, and in gathering information about compliance with the AAMC guidelines (Ehringhaus and Korn 2004; Ehringhaus et al. 2008).

Some empirical studies of disclosure about financial conflicts indicate that under some conditions, disclosure can exacerbate bias rather than reduce it. In experiments cited by the Institute of Medicine, those giving financial advice gave more biased information when they disclosed financial ties, knowing they were morally relieved by their disclosure, but those receiving the advice did not discount the bias to the same degree (Cain, Loewenstein, and Moore 2005, cited in Dana 2009). Jason Dana (2009) reviewed the pertinent psychological research for the 2009 Institute of Medicine study. Scientists and health professionals have strong professional norms that are not directly tested in these experiments, so the outcomes might be different in the context of science and clinical medicine and might differ from the results of the empirical surveys and experiments examined, but the results are nonetheless unsettling, indicating that disclosure is insufficient and may sometimes even create perverse incentives.

The experience of NIH intramural research staff since December 2003 illustrates both individual and institutional conflict-of-interest concerns. The *Los Angeles Times* ran a front-page feature by David Willman, "Stealth Merger: Drug Companies and Government Medical Research," on Pearl Harbor Day, 2003. The initial reaction was mainly denial that the problem was serious, along with accurate but defensive assurances that most NIH scientists have great integrity. Within months, a blue-ribbon panel that was assembled to look into the NIH's conflict-of-interest policies reported to a newly appointed NIH director, Elias Zerhouni (Metheny 2004). Members of Congress rejected the panel's recommendations as insufficient and excoriated the NIH for lax conflict-of-interest oversight. Dr. Zerhouni concluded that the NIH "failed to recognize how angry members of Congress and their staffs were over conflict of interest scandals at the agency" (Metheny 2004). This anger was reinforced by congressional investigations revealing that some NIH researchers failed to report or underreported their financial connections to private firms. Many of these cases could be explained by reporting errors or differences between the ways in which firms and the NIH were gathering data, but a few were obvious violations that reinforced concerns on Capitol Hill. Members of Congress had their distrust of the NIH reinforced, while NIH scientists and staff felt abused by the actions of a few outliers. These cases were nonetheless concrete evidence that scientists' disclosure was incomplete, as discovered when Congress got records directly from the pharmaceutical industry that were not reported by the NIH. Pressure mounted on the NIH to adopt simpler and more enforceable rules, with another front-page *Los Angeles Times* feature (Willman 2004) and other national coverage. The policy cascade culminated in new federal regulations that took effect for NIH and other employees of the Department of Health and Human Services on February 3, 2005 (Weiss 2005). When Dr. Zerhouni reported the new policies to NIH employees, the reception was unenthusiastic. In the *Washington Post*, the chief NIH bioethicist, Ezekiel Emanuel, was quoted as "fuming": "Even my secretary is going to have to sell her stock. How much sense does that make?" (Weiss 2005, A25). The rules nonetheless went into effect, with only mild changes.

The story then shifted to research institutions outside government, including academic health research centers. Much of the public attention on conflicts of interest traces to the activities of the Senate Finance Committee, and particularly the efforts of Senator Charles Grassley. Just as they had done for the NIH, committee staff gathered information from drug and device manufacturers and compared payments with the amounts reported by research institutions. Discrepancies and nondisclosure of financial ties between firms whose interests were connected to NIH-funded clinical research became major national scandals for investigators at Harvard (Joseph Biederman), Stanford (Alan Schatzberg), Emory (Charles B. Nemeroff), Washington University (Timothy R. Kuklo), George Washington University and National Public Radio (Frederick Goodwin), and other institutions. The roiling scandals elicited considerable policy attention. The April 2009 Institute of Medicine report cited sixteen policy reports written over eight years, between 2000 and 2008.

The Institute of Medicine's report noted that five states and the District of Columbia had passed laws requiring pharmaceutical manufacturers (and in some cases, device or biotechnology firms) to report their payments to physicians and other health professionals and organizations. Senators Grassley and Kohl introduced a bill, the Physician Payments Sunshine Act, in 2007, then reintroduced it early in the 111th Congress in 2009 (S. 301). The bill embodied the key recommendations of a June 2008 report to Congress from the Medicare Payment Advisory Commission. The bill had not come to a vote in the Senate as of November 2009, but Senate and House committees incorporated disclosure requirements into bills considered during the fall 2009 health care reform debate. Some observers linked disclosure to broader concerns about the rising cost of health care. As Natasha Singer (2009) wrote on the front page of the business section in the *New York Times*, "The [sunshine provisions'] targets are common business practices like drug company payments to doctors for speeches and consulting services, which have the potential to influence patient care and drive up the nation's medical bills."

The same week that the *New York Times* framed disclosure as part of the health care reform debate, the International Committee of Medical Journal Editors (2009b, 1896) released a "uniform format for disclosure of competing interests." The new form requests that authors disclose funding given directly for the published work as well as "all monies from sources with relevance to the submitted work," "long-term financial relationships that are now ended" but could still be the subject of criticism if not disclosed, and "financial relationships involving your spouse or partner or your children (under 18 years of age)" (International Committee of Medical Journal Editors 2009a, 1). The form also requests that authors "report any personal, professional, political, institutional, religious, or other associations that a reasonable reader would want to know about in relation to the submitted work." Critics objected to the breadth of the requested disclosure. Even Jerome Kassirer called the standard "a little excessive" (Armstrong 2009), and the industry newsletter *BioCentury* (2009) said that the new form was an "obvious and profound assault on privacy and liberty." Discussion of the new standards may raise the profile of conflicts of interest and disclosure higher.

The Roles of Academic Health Research

Academic institutions played at least three distinct roles in the national innovation system throughout the past century. They created an open science commons on which academic science and industry could draw, they sustained science not tied directly to profitable markets, and they were major sources of education and training for scientists (and managers) in both academia and industry. A fourth role has been added in the past two decades: fostering economic growth (Litan and Mitchell 2008). Each of these roles is relevant to thinking about the contending goals of academic research.

Patenting is only one sideshow in a complex production. Policies on publication, on data-sharing, on material transfer, and on personnel exchange and consulting are usually the main tools used by universities to maintain openness (Cohen and Walsh 2008), although attention to the specific terms of patent and licensing agreements is certainly important to ensuring the creation and dissemination of knowledge. Data from a 2002 survey study of university practices showed that even in the relatively well-settled area of publication—the core academic output—university-industry agreements differ widely. One-fourth of universities had clear agreements to protect their ownership and right to publish, one-half permitted some period of review or limited restrictions on publication rights, but one-fourth could be subject to corporate control of data, including publication, thus deviating from the standards of the International Committee of Medical Journal Editors (Schulman et al. 2002). In another study, investigators at institutions doing research under contract with industry did not have contract provisions ensuring data access that met editorial standards (Rettig 2000). And these are features of university-industry relationships that can be monitored, because agreements can be examined. Other practices that link companies directly to faculty and staff, such as consulting, speaking, and indirect research support, are much more difficult to monitor, because they do not necessarily involve the offices of sponsored (external) research or technology licensing offices.

In several areas, such as faculty consulting and signing of nondisclosure agreements between academics and companies, practices are monitored internally by some universities, but there are no clear-cut national standards and practices are diverse. Technology licensing offices are usually not in the loop, so this is a matter of general academic administration. Individual conflict of interest is thus mainly a matter for university faculty and staff, with oversight by administrators who cannot be sure they have all the information they should have.

The Growing Complexity of Science

Many players are involved in R&D. In the life sciences, small companies have added to the postwar mix of large pharmaceutical firms and academic research institutions, increasing the complexity of the national innovation system. Small firms vary in age from a few decades to brand new, and they vary greatly in size, focus, and style. Some of these are companies that grew out of university research, some are smaller and more nimble spin-offs from large firms. Until the 1980s, the classic model of industrial health research was the vertically integrated pharmaceutical firm that conducted drug-discovery research (while drawing on a public science base), funded development through toxicity testing and clinical trials, negotiated the complex Food and Drug Administration regulatory process, and distributed drugs through complex networks, with sales fomented by powerful marketing arms. Drug discovery is now widely distributed among firms of various sizes. Some organize clinical trials; some provide "platform technologies" for R&D; some offer R&D services or make instruments or write software; some occupy small therapeutic niches neglected by large pharmaceutical firms. There are even private, for-profit institutional review boards to perform ethical review.

The Industrialization of Clinical Research

Structures to keep scientific discovery and commercial development in a harmonious balance have not kept pace with the changes in health research (if, indeed, such structures ever existed, and if a balance was ever struck)

(Rettig 2000). Clinical research has become more industrialized and is now also seen as a business area with the potential for growth. Many conflicts of interest have arisen from this. In mid-1999, accusations surfaced regarding physicians purportedly paid to recruit patients for trials, the disclosure of financial interests of physician-investigators, and compensation of patients for trial participation. (Rettig 2000). The "poster child" of company abuse was the British pharmaceutical company Boots threatening action against University of California, San Francisco, researcher Betty Dong to block publication of a trial showing bioequivalence between the firm's formulation of thyroid hormone and other formulations (Wadman 1996). New York Attorney General Elliot Spitzer sued GlaxoSmithKline for suppressing the results of antidepressant clinical trials in children (Tansey 2004). To avoid suppression of clinical trial results, the National Library of Medicine has established a clinical trial registry, and editors of major medical journals have signaled their intent to publish results only of trials listed on that or another public registry (International Committee of Medical Journal Editors 2004).

According to Sheldon Krimsky (2003), there are three main areas where conflict of interest is most clearly a problem in clinical research. First, the financial interest of a clinical trial investigator in commercializing people's cell lines or genetic markers may conflict with his or her role as caregiver. Second, a physician could potentially put a patient in danger by deemphasizing certain risks, in the role of advising about trial participation or recruiting into trials (Krimsky 2003). Finally, researchers' financial interests may influence how a study is designed, whether results are reported, and how they are interpreted (Cohen, Nelson, and Walsh 2002).

The Private Value of Open Research

What is it that industries find valuable about academic research? Is it the patents they can license to others, the people they can hire, the prestige and credibility of academic experts, or the published information that their corporate scientists can draw on? It is all these things, but their importance is not equal and varies with context. The Carnegie-Mellon Survey of "inputs" to industrial R&D found that academic research had most of its impact through the "indirect" channels of publication, scientific meetings, and "open science"— that is, through a science commons that each company could draw on to develop products, and not just through formal mechanisms such as licensing of patented inventions from universities (Cohen, Nelson, and Walsh 2002).

The Carnegie-Mellon survey also found some other, distinctive aspects of pharmaceuticals. Publicly funded basic research was deemed to contribute more to pharmaceuticals than to most other industries. Patents and licenses were found to be important means to enable commercial development of discoveries made in academia, partly reflecting the fact that patent protection is stronger and more secure in drugs than in any other manufacturing industry. Start-up firms were also much more clearly tied to public research relevant to biotechnology and pharmaceuticals than in other industries. Federally funded academic research is thus a tide that raises all ships in the biotechnology and pharmaceutical sector.

Even within the narrow terms of fostering the growth of private commercial economic markets, it seems that, at the level of the innovation system as a whole, the value of the "open" aspects of publicly funded science probably exceeds any specific benefits of technology transfer through patenting and patent-licensing. More important, the value of "open" science seems considerable and likely to fly in the face of incentives to increase academic secrecy. While generally true, however, this observation does not help guide policy, because in any given case, social value may be gained by inducing private investment. Patents may not always be relevant, but when they are, they can be very important indeed. This is compounded by uncertainty about when and what to patent. At the time of discovery, it may well be difficult to predict how much subsequent investment is needed to make a new discovery useful. The scientist-inventors involved with the seminal recombinant DNA technologies at Stanford, the University of California, and Columbia were not at all certain that their patents were going to be useful, yet licenses on those patents raised $255 million for Stanford and the University of California (Reimers 1995; Hughes 2001; Feldman, Colaianni, and Liu 2007) and $790 million for Columbia (Colaianni and Cook-Deegan 2009). These are now held out as models of financially successful university technology licensing, but their commercial value at the time the deals were cut was not at all clear.

Where patents are decisive in inducing private R&D investment to translate a discovery into a product or service, secrecy, at least up to the time of filing patent applications, is essential to preserve worldwide rights. After filing a patent application, however, the justification for secrecy is considerably weaker—except to defend the commercial interests of industrial partners. That may be an important exception, but it is also one that can conflict directly with the value of open scientific disclosure, publication, and the academic mission of disseminating knowledge completely and rapidly. One remarkable void in the technology transfer literature is what academic institutions do about openness after patent applications are filed, aside from traditional publication. Much could be done to make data and materials available publicly at earlier dates, such as contributing DNA sequence data to public databases once a patent application is filed (National Research Council 1997; National Institutes of Health 1998; Cook-Deegan and McCormack 2001). Margo Bagley (2006) notes that disclosure is particularly important in academic research, and it can interact with incentives for secrecy in patent law, but there are also remedies that could promote both rapid scientific sharing and patent disclosure rules.

The research results that have attracted the most policy attention are so-called research tools (National Research Council 1997; National Institutes of Health 1998). Potential impediments to research were a major focus of a 2006 National Research Council report on intellectual property in genomics and proteomics. Many inventions arising in academic research will be both tools for further research and direct pathways to potential commercial products and services. The recombinant DNA patents noted above are examples of such "research tool" technologies. The debate about the patenting of genes turns in part on the dual role of most gene patents, as potentially covering not only end products (e.g., protein therapeutics resulting from the genes) but also research tools to study gene function, diagnostics to detect mutations, or components needed to study gene expression patterns as part of a "genome scan." Understanding a gene necessarily entails isolating it, making it, and using it (although not necessarily selling it).

By inducing investment in protein therapeutics and other end products, gene patents may be crucial to commercial development and subsequent health benefits. At the same time, only twenty thousand or so human genes exist to patent, and understanding their function is a compelling scientific priority. Jensen and Murray (2005) estimated that at least 20 percent of human genes were the subject of at least one U.S. patent claim, and Michael Hopkins et al. (2006) found more than sixteen thousand DNA sequence–based claims worldwide, the vast majority in the United States. If gene patents are used to block others from making and using genes in the laboratory, we are all much worse off. If patent holders exercised their full legal rights, gene patents would become a serious bottleneck to research. The same class of patents could thus be important in the classic sense of enabling private investment in an invention that requires substantial development costs after discovery, such as development of a therapeutic, and at the same time, if all patent rights were enforced to their fullest, could be a potent threat to research of broad import.

The conventions fostering the use of genes in research are not legal, but contingent on the forbearance of patent owners to permit research—a metastable and perhaps fragile situation. Many researchers believe they have a right to use a gene or any other patented invention for noncommercial purposes. Any illusion that U.S. law protects such academic research use evaporated in the face of the decision of the U.S. Court of Appeals for the Federal Circuit in *John M. J. Madey v. Duke University* (01-1567, 64 USPQ2d 1737 [Fed. Cir. 2002], Oct. 3), and in Europe, statutory research exemptions are only slightly broader. To date, forbearance has prevailed, and many technology licensing officers expect it to continue. They may prove right; they may be wrong.

It is possible to license such inventions so that academic research is unfettered but production for therapeutic use is subject to exclusive licensing, enabling broad research use while also inducing private R&D investment in therapeutics. The Cohen-Boyer (Stanford) and Axel (Columbia) patents, for example, were licensed with a de facto exemption from infringement for academic research. This was because Stanford and Columbia did not seek licenses from academic users, but only from commercial users. In another example of creative licensing, the University of Michigan handles U.S. licensing for a group of patents related to the cystic fibrosis transmembrane receptor, which it co-owns with the University of Toronto and Toronto's Hospital for Sick Children. Some of these patents are licensed nonexclusively for diagnostic use, resulting in many labs offering the test and earning modest royalties; some of the same patents have been licensed exclusively for gene transfer as a therapeutic, and some have been licensed on humanitarian terms, with no expectation of revenues, for treatment of diarrheal diseases in poor regions globally (Chandrasekharan et al. 2009). But such licensing is at the discretion of the patent administrator. These policies require foresight by licensing offices, to ensure that licensees cannot block academic research and other socially valuable noncommercial uses. The National Institutes of Health (2004a) proposed nonbinding guidelines to encourage licensing practices that preserve scientific freedom.

Social benefit from medical research depends on basic research finding its way into clinical application, and to the degree that such application entails commercial products and services and linkages between academic science and industrial development, university-industry relationships toward that end are a good thing. Yet clinical trialists who have a financial stake in the outcomes of their research have a strong and readily apparent conflict between their financial self-interest and the integrity of their science. Social benefit depends on ensuring that their professional behavior aligns with social benefit. That is why institutions are developing rules that set up a presumption that clinical researchers should not have a financial stake in companies whose products they are testing (Association of American Medical Colleges 2001; Institute of Medicine 2009). It is just such details about why and how incentives arise and what the social value of particular kinds of research is—and how these incentives align in different kinds of research—that need to guide policymaking.

Constituencies will contend with one another to adjust the rules and to get the attention of university administrators, the media, government officials, legislators, and the general public. As the importance of health research and the stakes involved in exercising power become more apparent, this will get more attention, and the attention may well breed more conflict. That is a common feature of political decision making.

Norms, Regulations, or Laws in Technology Licensing?

Universities recognize their public role and that it can conflict with maximizing revenue from inventions derived from federally funded research. Some make policy accordingly. The mission statement for technology licensing at Yale University (2006), for example, reads: "We use both financial and nonfinancial metrics to assess the value of an opportunity to society. Discoveries with high potential to improve the health or prosperity of the global community will be vigorously pursued irrespective of monetary gain to Yale." This makes clear that licensing policies take into account public interests, such as the global availability of essential medicines at reasonable cost. The statement says clearly that Yale will license to promote the use of a university invention even when such licensing might not maximize revenue for the university. MIT's licensing office (2006) has long stated its mission as "to benefit the public by moving results of MIT research into societal use via technology licensing, through a process which is consistent with academic principles, demonstrates a concern for the welfare of students and faculty, and conforms to the highest ethical standards"—a statement that implicitly subordinates revenue-maximizing to academic and social values. Such values are generally shared by academic technology licensing offices, but like other norms, this is not universal, and when norms alone guide policy, institutions will differ, sometimes markedly, in honoring them. Norms are flexible and can be nuanced; regulations are less flexible; laws are less flexible still. Moreover, norms matter only if there are standards and ways to judge compliance. Lack of transparency leaves only a "trust us" framework to do the work of enforcing norms. And it should be clear by now that investigative reporters, members of Congress, and nongovernment organizations are not apt to trust a system they believe has been corrupted. The flexibility of depending on norms is purchased at the price of heterogeneity and limited enforceability, as well as generally low credibility.

Universities' technology licensing mission statements and the shared norms among technology licensing professionals are thus a reason for optimism— because institutions can adjust norms to manage the new interests for public good, without need for the elaborate processes involved in legislation or regulation—but are also subject to the caveat that if shared norms are the main tools of policymaking, some institutions will not abide by them. There is limited capacity to monitor compliance in practice, and only "soft power" mechanisms are available for enforcing such norms. Achieving more uniformity tends to be slow and inconsistent and to be influenced by extreme cases of abuse that come to light. Cases of enlightened policy at some universities are balanced by other universities pursuing their private interests at obvious public expense. Columbia's effort to extend its Axel patents through backroom maneuvering on Capitol Hill was thwarted mainly because Public Citizen (2005) made the university's politicking public. A group of companies fought Columbia in court, the Public Patent Foundation called for a reexamination of the patent (Guzo 2004), and a judge's preliminary ruling led Columbia to sign a "covenant not to sue" for infringement of this patent (Columbia University 2004; Colaianni and Cook-Deegan 2009). In another case of abuse, Miami Children's Hospital exploited the families with Canavan disease whose contributions had made it possible to discover the gene and develop a diagnostic test, without remuneration (Gorner 2003; Hahn 2003). The hospital attempted to constrain the use of the diagnostic test by laboratories working with Ashkenazi Jewish organizations, provoking a lawsuit (*Greenberg v. Miami Children's Hospital,* 264 F. Supp. 2d 1064 [S.D. Fla. 2003]; Gorner 2003; Colaianni, Chandrasekharan, and Cook-Deegan 2009). While the legal interpretation is complex, assessing the *morality* (and wisdom) of the hospital's action is not a difficult case. When institutions file patents without informing stakeholders and impose conditions on inventions against the wishes of collaborators, something is amiss (Heaney et al. 2009). One perspective is that the system is working, given that the Florida case found remedy in the courts. And one way to design the system is to define boundaries by dealing with such outlier cases through litigation. Another perspective is that norms are insufficient and legislation is needed. The Physician Payments Sunshine Act is a move in that direction.

High-profile cases indicate that courts and legislative bodies will be among the places where policies governing the financial and social interests of academic research institutions are debated and may be decided. Unless norms of technology licensing are made more explicit and the system is made more transparent and accountable, abuses will invite stronger intervention by policymakers, in the form of regulation (subject to current law) and new legislation. Policies governing disclosure and management of conflict of interest are likewise on trial, both in the public media and, increasingly, in the courts. Absent meaningful enforcement of norms outside the courts, policy is likely to be formulated in reaction to grievances and cases of abuse, by both courts and legislatures reacting to scandal. Resolving contending interests will involve highly public conflict, at a cost to public trust in the research system.

The enormous growth of the health research enterprise suggests that opportunities for conflict may increase in frequency, will have serious consequences, and will sometimes involve academic research institutions. Just how to resolve the conflicts will depend, in part, on how academic institutions behave, whether they create credible norms, and whether they develop transparent, accountable procedures that instill public trust.

Conclusion

The fundamental problem facing academic health research is not that no one cares but that everyone cares very much, and increasingly so—as they should. The purpose of such research is to improve health, a prominent national and global goal. Research also directly contributes to economic growth. In most cases these goals align, but when they do not, which way and how far will academic institutions lean with respect to open scientific norms, maximization of public health, and financial gain?

Academic research centers are the largest and most conspicuous institutions that conduct publicly funded health research. They are the principal guardians of the science commons, on which the entire R&D ecosystem depends. Pharmaceutical, biotechnology, and medical device firms spend more on R&D than do academic research centers, and do a good deal of health research, but their work is far less public, their results are less widely shared, they do not play the same central role as the academic centers in training the research and management workforce, and they mainly (and properly, by design) pursue research that serves their own narrower, financial ends.

In 1980, the Bayh-Dole Act clarified national policy to encourage academic research institutions to work more closely with industry, reasoning that net social benefit would be increased by inducing private investment in the subsequent development of academic research discoveries. It worked in biotechnology and pharmaceuticals. The rise in innovation, however, grew not from just one policy, the Bayh-Dole Act, but from the convergence of several policies working in parallel: government funding of research, strengthening and broadening of intellectual property, tax policies that enabled institutional investors to fund risky ventures, and general economic policies to foster R&D investment and economic growth. It seems likely that the massive postwar infusion of public funds into research was the most powerful force, by creating a robust science commons on which science and industry could draw and inducing industrial investment in development. The massive increase in scale of health research has, in turn, made it a larger element of the national economy. This has drawn attention to the secondary effects of incentives to foster academic-industrial collaboration, including concern about conflicts of interest, both individual and institutional.

Several features that distinguish academic health research and contribute to its social value can be identified:

- *Openness.* If knowledge, data, and materials are widely shared, network efficiencies can take hold. Many players can draw on a science commons, even without central coordination (Benckler 2002). Disparate components of the knowledge economy gain access to more of their most important input—information—and can use state-of-the art tools and methods.
- *Pursuit of knowledge as an end,* which accounts for only a portion of academic research but is a portion unique to the public sector.
- *Science and technology not coupled to marketable products,* but highly relevant to public health, social policy, and other practical uses.
- *Education and training* of future workers—not just more researchers, but also industrial personnel in management and R&D.
- *Production* of inventions, data, and materials useful to industry.

The enormous growth of the scale and scope of health research suggests several major conclusions that bear on conflict of interest in academic health research:

- Funding for health research has increased spectacularly in both the public and private sectors.
- Increased funding means more research.
- More research means more intellectual property will be created.
- Industrial innovation for health is demonstrably more dependent on academic research than is innovation in other, even "high-technology," sectors.
- Intellectual property rights, and patents in particular, are generally more important in pharmaceuticals and medical biotechnology than in other sectors.

After World War II, health research became big science; it is now also big business. Managing contending social goals and financial interests will remain a prominent task at academic research institutions for the foreseeable future. More and better data are essential to guide future policy, but transparency is only a necessary and not a sufficient condition for the long-term health of the system, and even that necessary condition has not been achieved. In addition to information and openness, credible norms and practices must also be developed to ensure that research, particularly when it is publicly financed, reaches its intended social benefit. The predictable alternatives are scandal, litigation, regulation, and legislation.

NOTES

Epigraph. The Autobiography of Benjamin Franklin, pt. XVII, is available at http://odur.let.rug .nl/usa. Franklin goes on to note that others benefited from his inventions without his blessing, but also without his objection: "An ironmonger in London however, assuming a good deal of my pamphlet, and working it up into his own, and making some small changes in the machine, which rather hurt its operation, got a patent for it there, and made, as I was told, a little fortune by it. And this is not the only instance of patents taken out for my inventions by others, tho' not always with the same success, which I never contested, as having no desire of profiting by patents myself, and hating disputes. The use of these fireplaces in very many houses, both of this and the neighbouring colonies, has been, and is, a great saving of wood to the inhabitants." Note that even if Franklin had held a patent in Pennsylvania, it would not have mattered in London. Unless he could have patented his invention in England, Franklin is here claiming a generosity of spirit several thousand miles grander than its actual scope.

1. Henderson et al.'s interpretation of data on academic patents in general (Henderson, Jaffe, and Trajtenberg 1995) has been reanalyzed by others (Mowery et al. 1999, 2001), but the interpretive differences are not relevant to the point made here.

2. See, for example, testimony by Mark L. Rohrbaugh (2003), director of the Office of Technology Transfer, Office of the Director, National Institutes of Health, U.S. Department of Health and Human Services. Similar case studies were prepared by Holly Foskett, Office of Technology Licensing, Massachusetts General Hospital (personal communication), and by the NIH Office of Technology Transfer. A list is posted and individual case studies are available online (http://ott .od.nih.gov/about_nih/success_stories.aspx). Several chapters in the *IP Handbook of Best Practices*, produced by the Centre for Management of Intellectual Property in Health Research and Development, address global access to essential medical goods and services (www.iphand book.org).

REFERENCES

Armstrong, D. 2009. New conflict rules at medical journals. *Wall Street Journal*, Oct. 14.
Association of American Medical Colleges. 2001. *Protecting Subjects, Preserving Trust, Promoting Progress*. Vol. I. Washington, DC: Association of American Medical Colleges. www.aamc.org/ members/coitf.
————. 2002. *Protecting Subjects, Preserving Trust, Promoting Progress*. Vol. II. Washington, DC: Association of American Medical Colleges. www.aamc.org/members/coitf.
Association of University Technology Managers. 2006–9. Better World Project—reports. www .betterworldproject.org.
————. 2008. *AUTM Licensing Survey, FY 2007: Survey Summary*. Ed. R. T. Tieckelmann, R. Kordal, and D. Bostrom. Northbrook, IL: Association of University Technology Managers. www.autm .net.
Bagley, M. 2006. Academic discourse and proprietary rights: Putting patents in their proper place. *Boston College Law Review* 47 (1): 217–74.
Benckler, Y. 2002. Coase's Penguin, or, Linux and *The Nature of the Firm*. *Yale Law Review* 112 (3): 369–447.
BioCentury. 2009. Conscientious objection. *BioCentury: The Bernstein Report on BioBusiness*. www.biocentury.com.
Blumenthal, D., E. G. Campbell, M. Gokhale, R. Yucel, B. Clarridge, S. Hilgartner, and N. A. Holtz-man. 2006. Data withholding in genetics and other life sciences: Prevalences and predictors. *Academic Medicine* 81 (Feb.): 137–45.
Boyd, E. A., S. Lipton, and L. A. Bero. 2004. Implementation of financial disclosure policies to manage conflicts of interest. *Health Affairs* 23 (Mar./Apr.): 206–14.
Cain, D. M., G. Lowenstein, and D. A. Moore. 2005. The dirt on coming clean: Perverse effects of disclosing conflicts of interest. *Journal of Legal Studies* 34 (Jan.): 1–25.
Campbell, E. G., and E. Bendavid. 2003. Data-sharing and data-withholding in genetics and the life sciences: Results of a national survey of technology transfer officers. *Journal of Health Care Law and Policy* 6 (2): 241–55.

Campbell, E. G., B. R. Clarridge, M. Gokhale, L. Birenbaum, S. Hilgartner, N. A. Holtzman, and D. Blumenthal. 2002. Data withholding in academic genetics: Evidence from a national survey. *JAMA* 287 (4): 473–80.

Chandrasekharan, S., T. James, C. Heaney, C. Conover, and R. Cook-Deegan. 2009. Impact of gene patents and licensing practices on access to genetic testing for cystic fibrosis. In *Compendium of Case Studies on the Impact of Gene Patents and Licensing Practices on Access to Genetic Testing*. Prepared for the Secretary's Advisory Committee on Genetics, Health and Society. Washington, DC: National Institutes of Health. http://oba.od.nih.gov/SACGHS/sacghs_home.html.

Cockburn, I., and R. Henderson. 1996. Public-private interaction in pharmaceutical research. *Proceedings of the National Academy of Sciences of the United States of America* 93 (23): 12725–30.

Cohen, W. M., R. R. Nelson, and J. P. Walsh. 2002. Links and impacts: The influence of public research on industrial R&D. *Management Science* 48 (Jan. 1): 1–23.

Cohen, W. M., and J. P. Walsh. 2008. Real impediments to academic biomedical research. *Innovation Policy and the Economy* 8:1–30.

Colaianni, A., S. Chandrasekharan, and R. Cook-Deegan. 2009. Impact of gene patents and licensing practices on access to genetic testing and carrier screening for Tay-Sachs and Canavan disease. In *Compendium of Case Studies on the Impact of Gene Patents and Licensing Practices on Access to Genetic Testing*. Prepared for the Secretary's Advisory Committee on Genetics, Health and Society. Washington, DC: National Institutes of Health. http://oba.od.nih.gov/SACGHS/sacghs_home.html.

Colaianni, A., and R. Cook-Deegan. 2009. Columbia University's Axel patents: Technology transfer and implications for the Bayh-Dole Act. *Milbank Quarterly* 87 (3): 683–715.

Columbia University. 2004. Covenant not to sue for infringement of U.S. Patent 6,455,275 in the Federal District Court of Massachusetts, MDL No. 1592, Oct. 12. www.pubpat.org.

Comroe, J. H., and R. D. Dripps. 1976. Scientific basis for support of biomedical science. *Science* 192 (4235): 1105–11.

———. 1977. *The Top Ten Clinical Advances in Cardiovascular-Pulmonary Medicine and Surgery between 1945 and 1975: How They Came About*. Washington, DC: Government Printing Office.

Cook-Deegan, R. M., and S. J. McCormack. 2001. Patents, secrecy and DNA. *Science* 293 (July 13): 217.

Cook-Deegan, R., and M. McGeary. 2006. The jewel in the federal crown? History, politics, and the National Institutes of Health. In *History and Health Policy in the United States: Putting the Past Back In*, ed. R. A. Stevens, C. E. Rosenberg, and L. R. Burns, 176–201. New Brunswick, NJ: Rutgers University Press.

Dana, J. 2009. Appendix D: How psychological research can inform policies for dealing with conflicts of interest in medicine. In *Conflict of Interest in Medical Research, Education, and Practice*, ed. B. Lo and M. J. Field. Washington, DC: National Academies Press.

Davis, J. 2003. Patent criteria and scope. Paper presented at the meeting Science and Intellectual Property in the Public Interest, American Association for the Advancement of Science, Washington, DC.

Dustira, A. 1992. The funding of basic and clinical biomedical research. In *Biomedical Research: Collaboration and Conflict of Interest*, ed. R. J. Porter and T. E. Malone. Baltimore: Johns Hopkins University Press.

Ehringhaus, S., and D. Korn. 2004. *U.S. Medical School Policies on Individual Financial Conflicts of Interest: Results of an AAMC Survey.* Washington, DC: Association of American Medical Colleges.

Ehringhaus, S. H., J. S. Weissman, J. L. Sears, S. D. Goold, S. Feibelmann, and E. G. Campbell. 2008. Responses of medical schools to institutional conflicts of interest. *JAMA* 299 (6): 665–71.

Feldman, M., A. Colaianni, and K. Liu. 2007. Lessons from the commercialization of the Cohen-Boyer patents: The Stanford University licensing program. In *Intellectual Property Management in Health and Agricultural Innovation: A Handbook of Best Practices,* ed. A. Krattiger, R. T. Mahoney, L. Nelsen, et al., 1797–1808. Davis, CA: PIPRA.

———. Forthcoming. Commercializing Cohen-Boyer 1980–1997. *Research Policy.*

Gambardella, A. 1995. *Science and Innovation: The U.S. Pharmaceutical Industry during the 1980s.* New York: Cambridge University Press.

Gardner, C., and C. Garner 2004. Technology licensing to nontraditional partners: Nonprofit health product development organizations for better global health. *Journal of the Association of University Technology Managers* 16 (Summer): 29–42.

Ginzburg, E., and A. Dutka. 1989. *The Financing of Biomedical Research.* Baltimore: Johns Hopkins University Press.

Global Forum for Health Research. 2001. *Monitoring Resource Flows for Health Research, 2001.* Geneva: Global Forum for Health Research.

———. 2008. *Monitoring Financial Flows for Health Research, 2008.* Geneva: Global Forum for Health Research.

Goozner, M. 2004. *Unrevealed: Nondisclosure of Conflicts of Interest in Four Leading Medical and Scientific Journals.* Washington, DC: Center for Science in the Public Interest.

Gorner, P. 2003. Court allows suit on use of dead kids' DNA for patent. *Chicago Tribune,* June 8.

Guzo, D. 2004. Order granting ex parte re-examination of U.S. Patent 6,455,275, Application/Control number 90/006,953, U.S. Patent and Trademark Office, filed May 6.

Hahn, L. 2003. Owning a piece of Jonathan. *Chicago Magazine,* May: 83–87, 104–8.

Heaney, C., J. Carbone, R. Gold, T. Bubela, C. M. Holman, A. Colaianni, T. Lewis, and R. Cook-Deegan. 2009. The perils of taking property too far. *Stanford Journal of Law, Science and Policy* 1:46–64.

Henderson, R., A. Jaffe, and M. Trajtenberg. 1995. *Universities as a Source of Commercial Technology: A Detailed Analysis of University Patenting, 1965–1988.* Cambridge, MA: National Bureau of Economic Research.

Hopkins, M. M., S. Mahdi, S. M. Thomas, and P. Patel. 2006. *The Patenting of Human DNA: Global Trends in Public and Private Sector Activity (the PATGEN Project).* Final report to the 6th Framework Programme, European Commission. Falmer, UK: Science and Technology Policy Research, University of Sussex.

Hughes, S. S. 2001. The first major patent in biotechnology and the commercialization of molecular biology, 1974–1980. *Isis* 92 (3): 541–75.

Illinois Institute of Technology Research Institute. 1968. *Technology in Retrospect and Critical Events in Science.* Chicago: Illinois Institute of Technology.

Institute of Medicine. 1990. *Funding Health Sciences Research, a Strategy to Restore Balance.* Ed. B. Lo and M. J. Fields. Washington, DC: National Academies Press.

————. 2009. *Conflict of Interest in Medical Research, Education, and Practice.* Washington, DC: National Academies Press.

International Committee of Medical Journal Editors. 2004. Clinical trial registration, a statement of the International Committee of Medical Journal Editors. *Lancet* 364 (Sept. 11): 911–12.

————. 2009a. ICMJE uniform disclosure form for potential conflicts of interest. www.icmje.org.

————. 2009b. Uniform format for disclosure of competing interests in ICMJE journals. *New England Journal of Medicine* 361 (19): 1896–97.

International Expert Group on Biotechnology, Innovation and Intellectual Property. 2008. *Toward a New Era in Intellectual Property: From Confrontation to Negotiation.* Montreal: International Expert Group on Biotechnology, Innovation and Intellectual Property. www.theinno vationpartnership.org.

Jankowski, J. E. 1999. Trends in academic research spending, alliances, and commercialization. *Journal of Technology Transfer* 24 (1):55–68.

Jensen, K., and F. Murray. 2005. Intellectual property landscape of the human genome. *Science* 310 (Oct. 14): 239–40.

Kassirer, J. 2004. *On the Take: How Medicine's Complicity with Big Business Can Endanger Your Health.* New York: Oxford University Press.

Krimsky, S. 2003. *Science in the Private Interest: Has the Lure of Profits Corrupted Biomedical Research?* Oxford: Rowman & Littlefield.

Lei, Z., R. Juneja, and B. D. Wright. 2009. Patents versus patenting: Implications of intellectual property protection for biological research. *Nature Biotechnology* 27 (Jan.): 36–40.

Lipton, S., E. A. Boyd, and L. A. Bero. 2004. Conflicts of interest in academic research: Policies, processes, and attitudes. *Accountability in Research* 11 (2): 83–102.

Litan, R. E., and L. Mitchell. 2008. Should universities be agents of economic development? In *The Future of the Research University,* 123–38. Kansas City, MO: Ewing Merrill Kauffman Foundation.

Lowe, R. A., and S. K. Quick. 2004. Measuring the impact of university technology transfer: A guide to methodologies, data needs, and sources. *Journal of the Association of University Technology Managers* 16 (Summer): 43–59.

Malakoff, D. 2004. NIH roils academe with advice on licensing DNA patents. *Science* 303 (Mar. 19): 1757–58.

Mansfield, E. 1995. Academic research underlying industrial innovations: Sources, characteristics, and financing. *Review of Economics and Statistics* 77 (Feb.): 55–65.

Medicare Payment Advisory Commission. 2008. Public reporting of physicians' financial relationships. In *Report to Congress: Reforming the Delivery System.* Washington, DC: Government Printing Office.

Merton, R. K. 1973 [1942]. The normative structure of science. In *The Sociology of Science: Theoretical and Empirical Investigations,* ed. R. K. Merton, 267–80. Chicago: University of Chicago Press.

Metheny, B. 2004. Proactive NIH has worked with Congress to find common ground on conflicts of interest. *Washington Fax,* Nov. 11.

MIT, Technology Licensing Office. 2006. Our mission. http://web.mit.edu/tlo.

Mowery, D., R. R. Nelson, B. N. Sampat, and A. Ziedonis. 1999. The effects of the Bayh-Dole Act on U.S. university research and technology transfer. In *Industrializing Knowledge*, ed. L. Branscomb. Cambridge, MA: MIT Press.

———. 2001. The growth of patenting and licensing by U.S. universities: An assessment of the Bayh-Dole Act of 1980. *Research Policy* 30 (1): 99–119.

———. 2004. *Ivory Tower and Industrial Innovation: University-Industrial Technology Transfer before and after the Bayh-Dole Act.* Stanford, CA: Stanford Business Press.

Narin, F., and D. Olivastro. 1992. Status report: Linkage between technology and science. *Research Policy* 21 (3): 237–49.

Narin, F., and R. P. Rozek.1988. Bibliometric analysis of U.S. pharmaceutical industry research performance. *Research Policy* 17 (3): 139–54.

National Academy of Sciences. 2003. Beyond discovery. www.beyonddiscovery.org.

National Institutes of Health. 1998. *Report of the NIH Working Group on Research Tools.* Bethesda, MD: National Institutes of Health. www.nih.gov/news/researchtools.

———. 2004a. Best practices for the licensing of genomic inventions. *Federal Register* 69 (Nov. 19): 67747–48.

———. 2004b. *Report of the National Institutes of Health Blue Ribbon Panel on Conflicts of Interest.* Bethesda, MD: National Institutes of Health. www.nih.gov/about/ethics_COI_panelreport .pdf.

———. 2009a. The NIH almanac: Appropriations. www.nih.gov/about/almanac.

———. 2009b. Summary of the FY 2010 president's budget. http://officeofbudget.od.nih.gov.

National Research Council. 1995. *Allocating Federal Funds for Science and Technology.* Ed. S. A. Merrill, and A. M. Mazza. Washington, DC: National Academies Press.

———. 1997. *Intellectual Property Rights and Research Tools in Molecular Biology.* Washington, DC: National Academies Press.

———. 2006. *Reaping the Benefits of Genomic and Proteomic Research: Intellectual Property Rights, Innovation, and Public Health.* Washington, DC: National Academies Press.

National Science Foundation, Division of Science Resources Studies. 1999. *Federal R&D Funding by Budget Function: Fiscal Years 1998–2000.* Arlington, VA: National Science Foundation. www.nsf.gov/statistics/fedbudget.

———. 2001a. *Federal R&D Funding by Budget Function: Fiscal Years 1999–2001.* Arlington, VA: National Science Foundation. www.nsf.gov/statistics/fedbudget.

———. 2001b. *Federal R&D Funding by Budget Function: Fiscal Years 2000–2002.* Arlington, VA: National Science Foundation. www.nsf.gov/statistics/fedbudget.

———. 2002. *Federal R&D Funding by Budget Function: Fiscal Years 2001–03.* Arlington, VA: National Science Foundation. www.nsf.gov/statistics/fedbudget.

———. 2004a. *Federal R&D Funding by Budget Function: Fiscal Years 2002–04.* Arlington, VA: National Science Foundation. www.nsf.gov/statistics/fedbudget.

———. 2004b. *Federal R&D Funding by Budget Function: Fiscal Years 2003–05.* Arlington, VA: National Science Foundation. www.nsf.gov/statistics/fedbudget.

———. 2006a. *Federal R&D Funding by Budget Function: Fiscal Years 2004–06.* Arlington, VA: National Science Foundation. www.nsf.gov/statistics/fedbudget.

———. 2006b. *Federal R&D Funding by Budget Function: Fiscal Years 2005–07.* Arlington, VA: National Science Foundation. www.nsf.gov/statistics/fedbudget.

———. 2007. *Federal R&D Funding by Budget Function: Fiscal Years 2006–08.* Arlington, VA: National Science Foundation. www.nsf.gov/statistics/fedbudget.

———. 2008. *Federal R&D Funding by Budget Function: Fiscal Years 2007–09.* Arlington, VA: National Science Foundation. www.nsf.gov/statistics/fedbudget.

Office of Management and Budget. 2009. *Table 10.1—Gross Domestic Product and Deflators Used in the Historical Tables: 1940–2014.* Washington, DC: Office of Management and Budget. www .whitehouse.gov/omb/budget/Historicals.

Organization for Economic Cooperation and Development. 2008. OECD health data, 2008— frequently requested data. www.irdes.org/EspaceAnglais/home.html.

Pharmaceutical Research and Manufacturers of America. 2009. *Pharmaceutical Industry Profile 2009.* Washington, DC: Pharmaceutical Research and Manufacturers of America. www .phrma.org.

Pressman, L., and L. Walters. 2004. Presentations to Association of University Technology Managers annual meeting, San Antonio, TX, Mar.

Public Citizen. 2005. Columbia University patent extension would cost consumers, open floodgates for more special deals: Groups urge senators to remove rider added secretly to appropriations bill. www.citizen.org.

Rai, A. K., and R. S. Eisenberg. 2003. Bayh-Dole reform and the progress of biomedicine. *Law and Contemporary Problems* 66 (Spring): 289–314.

Reimers, N. 1995. Tiger by the tail. *Journal of the Association of University Technology Managers* 7 (1): 14–27 (orig. pub. *CHEMTECH* [American Chemical Society] 17, no. 8 [1987]: 464–71).

Rettig, R. 2000. The industrialization of clinical research. *Health Affairs* 19 (2): 129–46.

Rohrbaugh, M. L. 2003. NIH: Moving research from the bench to the bedside. Testimony before the Subcommittee on Health, Committee on Energy and Commerce, United States House of Representatives. July 10. www.ott.nih.gov.

Rosenfeld, S. C. 1988. Sharing of research results in a federally sponsored gene mapping project. *Rutgers Computer and Technology Law Journal* 14 (2): 211–58.

Schulman, K. A., D. M. Seils, J. W. Timbie, J. Sugarman, L. Dame, K. Weinfurt, D. B. Mark, and R. M. Califf. 2002. A national survey of provisions in clinical-trial agreements between medical schools and industry sponsors. *New England Journal of Medicine* 347 (17): 1335–41.

Singer, N. 2009. Health bills aim a light on doctors' conflicts. *New York Times,* Nov. 4.

Smith, B. L. 1990. *American Science Policy since World War II.* Washington, DC: Brookings Institution.

So, A. D., B. N. Sampat, A. K. Rai, R. Cook-Deegan, J. H. Reichman, R. Weissman, and A. Kapczynski. 2009. Is Bayh-Dole good for developing countries? Lessons from the US experience. *PLoS Biology* 6 (Oct.): 2078–84.

Stevens, A. 2004. The enactment of Bayh-Dole. *Journal of Technology Transfer* 29 (Jan.): 93–99.

Tansey, B. 2004. Glaxo settles fraud suit. *San Francisco Chronicle,* Aug. 27.

Thursby, J. G., and M. C. Thursby. 2007. University licensing. *Oxford Review of Economic Policy* 23 (Winter): 620–39.

U.S. Congress, Office of Technology Assessment. 1984. *Commercial Biotechnology: An International Analysis.* Washington, DC: Government Printing Office. www.princeton.edu/~ota/.

———. 1991. *Biotechnology in a Global Economy.* Washington, DC: Government Printing Office. www.princeton.edu/~ota/.

U.S. Department of Health, Education and Welfare. 1978. The patenting of recombinant DNA research inventions developed under DHEW support. *Recombinant DNA Technical Bulletin* 1 (2): 23–28.

U.S. Department of Health and Human Services. 2005. 5 CFR 5501 and 5502: Supplemental standards of ethical conduct and financial disclosure for employees of the Department of Health and Human Services. *Federal Register* 70 (Feb. 3): 5543–65.

U.S. Department of Health and Human Services, Office of the Inspector General. 1994. *Underreporting Federal Involvement in New Technologies at Scripps Research Institute.* Washington, DC: Department of Health and Human Services, Inspector General.

———. 1995. *NIH Oversight of Extramural Research Inventions.* Washington, DC: Department of Health and Human Services, Inspector General.

U.S. General Accounting Office. 1999. *Technology Transfer: Reporting Requirements for Federally Sponsored Inventions Need Revision.* Washington, DC: General Accounting Office.

Wadman, M. 1996. Drug company "suppressed" publication of research. *Nature* 381 (May 2): 4.

Walsh, J. P., W. M. Cohen, and C. Cho. 2007. Where excludability matters: Material versus intellectual property in academic biomedical research. *Research Policy* 36 (Oct.): 1184–1203.

Weinfurt, K. P., M. A. Dinan, J. S. Allsbrook, J. Y. Friedman, M. A. Hall, K. A. Schulman, and J. Sugarman. 2006. Policies of academic medical centers for disclosing financial conflicts of interest to potential research participants. *Academic Medicine* 81 (Feb.): 113–18.

Weiss, R. 2005. NIH workers angered by new ethics rules. *Washington Post*, Feb. 3.

Willman, D. 2003. Stealth merger: Drug companies and government medical research. *Los Angeles Times*, Dec. 7.

———. 2004. The National Institutes of Health: Public servant or private marketer? *Los Angeles Times*, Dec. 22.

———. 2005. NIH chief calls for ethics summit. *Los Angeles Times*, Feb. 12.

Wilson, C. 2003. Miami judge: Group can sue over gene researcher's patent on testing. *Miami Herald Tribune*, June 4.

Yale University, Office of Cooperative Research. 2006. About Yale OCR. www.yale.edu/ocr.

Zinner, D. E., D. Bjankovic, B. Clarridge, D. Blumenthal, and E. G. Campbell. 2009. Participation of academic scientists in relationships with industry. *Health Affairs* 28 (Nov./Dec.): 1815–25.

CHAPTER 3

From Conflict to Confluence of Interest

The Coevolution of Academic Entrepreneurship and Intellectual Property Rights

HENRY ETZKOWITZ, PH.D.

The university, an institution of medieval provenance for the conservation and dissemination of knowledge, is increasingly viewed as providing an ideal infrastructure for the generation, prototyping, and transfer of new technologies. The global objective of innovation policy is to weave a seamless web from laboratory to market, from bench to bedside, and from societal needs to the meandering stream of basic research. A panoply of interface mechanisms have been invented, such as the technology transfer office, to seek out inventions internally, patent and license them externally, assist in the adjudication of disputes over inventions, and help inventors identify resources to spin off firms. Incubator programs to assist in the formation of firms and venture capital initiatives to finance them have become an overlay on the technology transfer offices as the university acts as entrepreneur. Teaching and research missions are realigned and expanded, as entrepreneurship becomes part of the curriculum and as faculty involvement in start-ups inspires new research.

A shift is also under way in the entrepreneurial academic format, from patenting and licensing to existing firms toward formation of new firms based on academic-generated intellectual property. The Association of University Technology Managers (2000) identified $1.46 billion in earnings from patent licenses in FY 2000 and the formation of 3,376 firms based on technology licensed from universities between 1980 and 2000. As a close observer put it, "It is hard to point to a robust regional economy that is not in some sense anchored by a major research university or two" (L. Tornatzky, quoted in Schmidt 2001). Academic-industry relationships are transformed from a focus on consulting relationships and research partnerships with the research and development units of established firms, as science-based firms increasingly emerge from academia in incubator facilities on campus and locate in science parks adjacent to campus.

The patent mechanism has been used as a means of balancing dissemination and capitalization of knowledge, with regulation of commercialization tasks through university technology transfer offices. Resolution of academic conflicts of interest is based on two principles: (1) complementarity of activities—that is, whether the new activity enhances an older one; and (2) an agreed-upon division of time between the new and established tasks. The first issue is conceptualized as transition from conflict to confluence of interest, while the second relates to conflict of obligation and its regulation. When an external task is internalized, conflicts of interest may be resolved or at least moderated. The recent internalization of transfer capabilities at the university reflects an expansion of academic mission, legitimated by federal law. The establishment of generous leave policies encourages the relatively smooth externalization of firm-formation projects, moderating earlier disputes about time commitment.

When the primary purpose of the university was to train students, role definition was straightforward. When research became an academic mission as well, issues of conflict of interest were raised. Could a professor carry out the duties as teacher if attention was also directed to research? Despite persisting tensions, the overall assessment is that each role enhances the other. However, the fundamental issue of balancing multiple roles and making them complementary has reemerged as professors have become entrepreneurs. This chapter analyzes the coevolution of the university and the patent system as a case study in the resolution of conflicts of interest and obligation in the emerging "third academic mission": to contribute to economic and social development.

Scientific Exceptionalism?

Financial conflict appeared at the birth of modern science in the seventeenth century, as a few members of the Royal Society, such as Robert Hooke, sought income from their inventions (Merton 1938). In the late nineteenth century, MIT (the Massachusetts Institute of Technology) hired consulting professors to jump-start research at what was then an engineering teaching college (Etzkowitz 2002). These professors continued consulting despite collegial advice to keep to teaching, arguing that bringing real-world problems into the classroom made them better teachers. A similar issue arose at Stanford during the same era, as faculty researchers were charged with conflicts of interest. The time-commitment issue was resolved at MIT by invention of the "one-fifth rule" that spread throughout U.S. academia, allowing consultation activities one day a week and thus turning conflict into a confluence of interest; the teaching-versus-research issue was resolved through normative change, the acceptance of research as a university mission.

Conflict of interest, in the classic sense, exists when an individual in an organization has an external involvement that interferes with his or her professional responsibilities. A second type of conflict arises from a contradiction between enacting two roles in an organization. These two types of conflict, of interest and obligation, are expressed in academia as (1) potential effects of an external involvement on impartial judgment and (2) enacting two, simultaneous roles whose time or other requirements clash (Etzkowitz 1996). The first type has been most clearly expressed within government to denote officials' use of the powers of their office to confer benefits on themselves from external sources. The second type, the potential for conflict of interest from dual involvements, has been especially strongly articulated in the legal profession (Shapiro 2002). In taking on a new client, an attorney must determine whether he or she already represents a client with an opposing interest. Such a potential conflict does not necessarily preclude representation, but it does indicate the need to inform both parties of the situation.

Similarly, in universities, recognition of existing conflicts of interest has largely superseded the tendency to deny their existence, which derives from the often deeply held conviction that science is a process of creating knowledge that excludes social and political influences. In response to the Nazi subversion of science to conform to its ideological and political objectives, sociologist Robert Merton codified the "norms of science" in the early 1940s (Merton 1973 [1942]). His spirited response to this infamous attack on science and on scientists of Jewish origin was subsequently abstracted from the social and political context of its origin and reified into an autonomous theory of knowledge production.

On the one hand, proponents of the Mertonian norms expected science to be free of the fraud, self-dealing, and other forms of socially negative and ethically proscribed behavior commonly recognized as requiring regulation even in the classic professions. On the other hand, the uses of science were held to be separate from the creation of scientific knowledge, with separate and divergent roles and organizations and with different personnel and institutional frameworks. Both of these assumptions have been challenged in recent decades.

Significant cases of fraud, such as Hwang Woo-suk's faked data in support of the claim to have cloned embryonic stem cells, and other instances pressured by the rewards of priority research, have given rise to a sociology of "scientific deviance," and penalties have been applied to wrongdoers (Bechtel, 1985, 2000; Cyranowski, 2006). Generation of firms such as Genentech and Google, with academic input and assistance, has provided grist for the thesis of "academic capitalism" as a vitiating of academic integrity and mission (Slaughter and Rhodes 2004). Some observers conflate these trends and view scientific fraud and commodification of knowledge as virtually one and the same (Washburn 2005). I argue here, to the contrary, that direct academic involvement in translating knowledge into use is consistent with the traditional high purpose of universities and merely takes it to a new level and domain.

From the Research to the Entrepreneurial University

The "capitalization of knowledge" is at the heart of a new mission for the university, linking universities more tightly to users of knowledge and establishing the university as an economic actor in its own right. Academic institutions proceed through the stages and phases of mission change at different rates, without an inherent linear progression: a teaching institution—such as Babson College, Massachusetts—may move directly to play an entrepreneurial role and then take up a research mission. Nevertheless, for most institutions there is a continuous common progression, with teaching colleges (such as Albany State) upgrading to become research universities (the University at Albany) and then further expanding (at Albany, through establishment of the College of Nanoscale Science and Engineering) to become entrepreneurial universities.

In a reverse linear progression, land-grant schools move into basic research, as agricultural research funding for solving regional farming problems remains static but basic research funds, especially in health care, increase—encouraging land-grant schools to compete for these basic research funds from the National Institutes of Health and to expand their research activities in biotechnology. Nevertheless, previous functions persist. For example, the University of California, Berkeley, a leading research university, has an agricultural extension officer in the School of Natural Resources, reflecting its land-grant heritage—although, most likely, few contemporary Berkeley faculty are aware of the campus's early-twentieth-century preeminence in semiarid agriculture (Florence 2007). Even fewer would know that a county agent is still affiliated to the school, at the insistence of agricultural interests that want to retain an association with the University of California's leading campus.

As universities take on new missions, they develop organizational innovations and undergo normative change to integrate new tasks with old. Thus, the research group integrates training with advancement of knowledge, as student members, at various levels, learn from their peers and from those at higher and lower levels in the group, as well as from the principal investigator. Similarly, the incubator, an organizational innovation imported from industry to transfer technology through firm-formation, has become a method of training a group of individuals to operate as a well-functioning unit in the academic setting. This has thus become part of the university's educational mission, extended from individuals to groups. Integration of the patent mechanism into academia as part of an economic-development mission for technology transfer also becomes part of the university's original purpose of disseminating knowledge, now through patent databases as well as through articles, books, and lectures.

The entrepreneurial university is the culmination of an academic transformation that started with the transformation from teaching college to research university: the first "academic revolution," the take-up of research as an academic mission from the mid nineteenth century (Jencks and Riesman 1968). A second revolution, combining teaching, research, and economic and social development, is currently under way. Successive academic revolutions have made the university a capacious organization with the ability to accomplish multiple missions simultaneously, in contrast to firms, which are periodically forced to narrow their focus and concentrate on a "core competency." The university, then, has evolved in the opposite direction, from single to multiple functions and from a focus on relationships among individuals (e.g., teachers and students, faculty and administrators) to an organizational mode of operation through research groups and centers.

An understanding of academic conflict of interest requires specification of the purpose of the academic institution and the nature and requirements of its roles. The changing relationship among university, industry, and government also factors into the analysis. The transition from the research to the entrepreneurial university intersects with transition of the government role from regulating separate institutional spheres to encouraging interactions among them—in this case, through revision of the patent law and other incentives.

A "triple helix" of university-industry-government interactions emerges as government-industry and university-industry links overlap (Etzkowitz 2008). Each institutional sphere, in addition to performing its traditional role, also "takes the role of the other," with government serving as a public venture capitalist, industry taking training to higher levels in company universities, and universities performing increasingly direct economic roles in translating research with technological implications into use. From a triple helix perspective, the appearance of conflicts of interest may be taken as a positive sign that a sclerotic system is becoming flexible and that people are taking creative steps, transcending their traditional roles, to put knowledge to use.

The University as Patentee

Early instances of technology transfer from academic research in pharmaceuticals have been identified at German universities, occurring in the seventeenth century (Gustin 1975). The professionalization of university technology transfer began with the establishment of the Research Corporation (RC), a not-for-profit entity set up in 1912 by Frederick Cottrell, a chemistry professor at the University of California, Berkeley, in response to the university's refusal to manage the intellectual property rights of a faculty inventor. RC assumed these rights at the initiative of the inventor, who turned them over as a founding endowment.[1] A national program for technology transfer sought inventions from universities across the United States and supported faculty research with the proceeds. The project took off when MIT decided against developing an internal professional transfer capacity, instead retaining RC as a compromise between faculty members highly involved in transfer and those opposed (Etzkowitz 2002).

On a parallel track, the University of Wisconsin, a land-grant foundation, developed a transfer capability in a legally independent foundation that nevertheless remained under university control (Apple 1989). The university was impelled to develop this capacity, having achieved several inventions with considerable market potential in the dairy and food supplement (vitamin) industries. The University of Toronto, a school with no previous interest in technology transfer, nevertheless patented and licensed the discovery by members of its staff of a means to produce insulin, to ensure its ethical manufacture (Bliss 1982). The university received royalties through its agreement with Eli Lilly, but this specific arrangement did not lead to a systematic technology transfer program at the time, because of the university's traditional academic culture.

During this early era, universities learned that there is a moral imperative to patent, to ensure both that the results of academic research are put to use and that the transfer is accomplished efficaciously and ethically. The university's technology transfer office is responsible for conducting "due diligence" in identifying partners and monitoring that agreements are followed. Moreover, the university has a responsibility to ensure its own financial health and stability by capturing a reasonable share of the revenues from the intellectual capital that it generates. The federal government recognized this objective in the Bayh-Dole Act of 1980.

A relatively few universities, including MIT and University of Wisconsin, had earlier accepted this mission, but they were viewed as anomalies. In the wake of passage of the 1980 law, research universities—starting with those with the highest levels of federal funding and then moving to less research-intensive schools—established at least a minimal technology transfer capability, typically by hiring industrial scientists familiar with a field in which the university had research strength with commercial potential. Although this step was typically taken to meet federal requirements, people in the technology transfer position took it seriously. Some were lucky and soon had a "big hit," such as the Axel patent on co-transformation of genes at Columbia University Medical School, leading to the rapid expansion of technology transfer at that university. Other schools, typically but not always the less research-intensive, were less fortunate and became stuck at levels of support inadequate to break out of failure mode.

There are two essential elements to academic technology transfer: (1) the ability to license technologies for which the university/inventor has applied for a patent, and (2) the ability to collaborate with the inventor of the technology to further develop it. The first of these two steps constitutes the actual transfer of the technology, but given the early stage of academic technology, it is often not worthwhile making the transfer unless the second option is also available and the cooperation of the inventor is already secured.

In fact, universities can choose to handle their patents in many different ways. On the one hand, universities striving for immediate income can license their inventions to large corporations with the ability to pay. On the other hand, taking a longer-term view, and either at their own initiative or at the behest of regional authorities concerned about local economic growth, universities can license to start-ups for equity instead of royalty income. This is especially the case for new start-ups that are tied to the region and are viewed both as an instrument of local economic growth and as long-term capital appreciation for the university, because equity in a successful firm can bring far greater returns than even the largest royalty stream from a patent license.

The unexpected scale of the earnings from Google transformed the Stanford University administration's expectations of technology transfer.[2] A quarter of a billion dollars plus held the potential for new buildings and programs, making possible initiatives orders of magnitude beyond supporting graduate students. The scale of the Google IPO (initial public stock offering) also led to a rethinking of transfer, especially within the Stanford Management Corporation that invests the university's endowment.[3] The Management Corporation viewed the more than $250 million that the university earned from its ownership of a small percentage of the equity in Google as a relative failure. The IPO had realized billions, but the university had gained only a small part of the earnings. The Management Corporation proposed that, in future, the university should make a modest investment in each new firm that its transfer office licensed, modestly but significantly increasing the university's share of equity.

The Origins of Academic Patenting

The patenting of inventions by research universities emerged as a byproduct of the transition of the university from an institution focused on teaching to one in which research is an important activity. The early proponents of making the university a site of original investigation were intent on pure science; the emphasis on research also occurred in medical and engineering schools, where the interest was more practical. Nevertheless, pure research could not be separated from invention, given that a useful device might unexpectedly emerge from the pursuit of knowledge for its own sake (Pupin 1923).

Universities explicitly committed to the practical exploitation of knowledge and inventions, of course, were more aware than others of the need to address issues of technology transfer, rather than assuming that it could take care of itself according to laissez-faire principles. The reputation of the university, its financial well-being, and even public health and safety were at stake.

As with other issues of university-industry relationships, such as the role of the university in regional development, the experience of MIT with patents is instructive. Given MIT's industrial mission and academic focus, the potential commercial value of its research was well recognized before the 1920s. But until the early 1930s, MIT followed a laissez-faire policy with respect to patents. Sometimes, members of the academic staff assigned the rights to take out patents to the institute; at other times, they retained the rights to themselves. There was rising concern, however, that if MIT did not take responsibility for the potential intellectual property that the school was generating, outsiders could tap into research results and patent them on their own behalf. Not only would this take away resources that the school could use to support itself (a concern that arose after MIT lost its funding from the State of Massachusetts), but the school's reputation could be tarnished if faulty products were marketed in the absence of quality control.

In response, President Compton appointed a committee in late 1931 to formulate a patent policy for MIT. The committee included both proponents and opponents of academic patenting. Compton charged the committee with the following tasks: "(1) To ensure that ambiguity in regard to questions of title shall be clarified within a reasonable period. (2) To ensure that the Institute is placed in a position to profit from its own developments in any case in which it may choose to do so, and thereby ensure a prompt realization to the public of the benefits of any such developments. (3) To sustain the interest and enthusiasm of the friends of the Institute where ever they may be placed" (MIT 1932). The charge itself presumed acceptance of an academic patent right (Etzkowitz 2002). Compton's objectives were twofold. He wanted to develop MIT into a scientific and technological university of great academic distinction (Lécuyer 1992). He also believed that advanced research could contribute directly to economic development and that the advancement and commercialization of research could each contribute to furthering the other.

Compton and his associates in the MIT administration sought academic distinction of a high and special kind, combining fundamental inquiry with practical use. Vannevar Bush (1970), a faculty member in electrical engineering, provided a model for the entrepreneurial academic who combines contribution to theoretical advance in his discipline with invention and commercialization of useful devices. Bush continually extrapolated theoretical and practical implications from any technology that he came across. He obtained many of his research ideas from his consulting practice, and his students would then work, under his supervision, on the academic implications. At times, new practical implications would emerge from these investigations.

Bush's experience exemplified Compton's goals for MIT. The final element, closing the loop, was to place these ideas into industrial use, either in existing firms or in new ones formed for the purpose. Bush (1970, 159) told the Temporary National Economic Commission that he had never directly made any money from a patent. "But indirectly is another matter, as they well understood. I was early a professor and also a consultant to industry. It was a salutary combination; it drew me out of the ivory tower and put life into my teaching, and it greatly helped the family budget." Through his college roommate, Laurence K. Marshall, Bush made the acquaintance of a group of Boston financiers, who invested in several companies that Bush helped organize when he was a consultant in the years after World War I. These companies included Spencer Thermostat, which eventually became part of Texas Instruments, and Raytheon (Bush 1970, 168).

As with the early controversy over consulting, the debate over patenting was resolved through compromise. Opponents of patenting argued that it would tarnish MIT's academic reputation to become involved in commercial pursuits and, further, that patents were costly to obtain, few would bring returns, and the school would probably lose money from the venture. These issues, as well as the belief that academic work, as a public good, should be freely available to all, are similar to those articulated by contemporary critics of academic patenting. However, MIT's mission to infuse the Boston region and local industry with new technology provided a basis to establish a process to scrutinize inventions for their commercial potential and seek partners to commercialize them. MIT also decided that it should not take on the marketing part of this business function directly, and it engaged RC to do so.

In addition to contributing to regional economic development, other considerations impelled universities to adopt patent policies. They needed to protect their reputations and ensure quality control of devices produced from their academic discoveries. If they took no action at all, other than publication, university laboratories would be left open to "vultures" in search of free useful knowledge that could be patented for their own financial benefit.

Patents taken out by persons who were not the inventors would result in knowledge discovered by academic scientists being made into the private property of persons or institutions who had no part in the discovery, which could be fatal to the health of patients and damage the reputation of the university, laying it open to legal action.

Such was the case at the University of Toronto Medical School, where Frederick Banting and Charles Best's discovery of insulin in 1921–22 led to a classic shift in stance toward academic patenting (Bliss 1982). The researchers had developed a treatment for diabetes, which drew intense interest from patients, their families, and the public in general, given the publicity about the research. Large profits, public health, and the reputation of the university were at stake. The Toronto case also raised a series of issues between university administrators and teachers and business firms, including the distribution of money earned and the propriety of ceding patent rights to a single firm. Putting contrary policy aside, the University of Toronto decided to acquire a patent on insulin, a much-demanded drug in extremely short supply. University administrators believed that by licensing the university's patent to a single reputable pharmaceutical firm, the Eli Lilly Company, quality control could be assured and revenue gained to support future research. The ethical rules to which the university was committed precluded personal gain from the patent. The university's alliance with Lilly enabled its researchers to translate findings into clinical practice quickly, ensuring credit for their discovery against other claimants.[4] Patenting was a useful mechanism both to divide credit for the discovery and to control the commercialization process to ensure that it took place in an orderly manner, under the control of the university.

The University of Wisconsin, a school strongly committed to research with a practical orientation, experienced the negative consequences of not properly protecting inventions produced by its faculty members. When Stephen Moulton Babcock invented a device for testing the quality of milk, several unscrupulous manufacturers marketed faulty equipment to farmers, representing it as the Babcock invention. Without patent protection, the university had no means of protecting itself or the public from the makers of these devices. Because of the publicity about the discovery at the university, the public held the school responsible for contaminated milk, even though the matter was out of its control. The university's reputation suffered from the commercialization of technology that did not perform as expected. Even though the university was involved only in the invention, with production left to others, the public expected the university to be responsible for the entire process and blamed it for products that did not work (Apple 1989).

Just as the University of Toronto patented to protect the quality of insulin production, so the University of Wisconsin suffered the consequences of not having control over an invention made on campus. In 1925, the University of Wisconsin formed a patent-management organization, the Wisconsin Alumni Research Foundation, to directly manage the intellectual property rights generated on campus for the financial benefit of the university and the economic benefit of the state, as well as to ensure careful manufacture. The funds generated from patent licensing allowed the university to develop its biological sciences disciplines to high distinction during the Depression years.

Before World War II, few academic scientists and engineers thought it was part of their task to generate commercially profitable results and to file a patent. This was thought to be a task for their counterparts in industry. Even an industrially oriented academic institution did not find patenting free of problems. MIT was aware of the negative reaction to the University of Wisconsin's policy in dealing with patents. In this instance, protection of local industries affected how a university used its patents. The University of Wisconsin refused to license vitamin D supplements to margarine manufacturers, in order to protect the economic interests of the state's dairy producers.

Nevertheless, this instance of "protectionism," for which the university was widely criticized, ultimately served more as a deterrent to universities' use of the patent system for this purpose than as a precedent. Indeed, MIT was mindful of the Wisconsin experience when it developed its patent policy. An MIT report (1936) found that "one educational Institution, which has derived a considerable income from one group of patents, has been severely criticized in scientific circles for its patent policy due to its method in handling the subject rather than to the mere fact that income is derived." MIT attempted to reconcile its 1861 charter, which gave it a special responsibility to combine academic goals of research and dissemination of knowledge, with assistance to industry.

The Impact of World War II

A patent system conceived to promote individual entrepreneurship was adapted to sustain organizational entrepreneurship, but by a different path than that followed by corporations, which subsumed 100 percent of the direct rewards, giving promotions and bonuses to employees based, in part, on invention success. Academic institutions, by contrast, shared a proportion of the rewards directly with faculty inventors—or it could be said that inventors shared the rewards with their schools. This is how universities interpreted the patent system, initially at a few schools such as MIT and Wisconsin and then more broadly. The potential for university technology transfer on a larger scale was an outcome of the increase in federal funding for academic research during and after World War II. The expectation was that this research would lead to manifold civilian uses in the postwar period, just as it had resulted in innovations in weaponry during the war. As government funds expanded the scale and scope of academic research, the potential for the patenting of research findings increased.

Before the war, patenting and licensing had largely been based on foundation, industry, and self-funded research. During the war, patent rights began to be generated on a large scale as a result of expanded federal research funding. As director of the wartime Office of Scientific Research and Development, Vannevar Bush (1970) arranged for the patenting of government-sponsored research. He was aware from his earlier experience at MIT that an expansion of research would generate intellectual property and that if conflicts were to be avoided, patents would have to be managed. Even during the war there was a view toward peacetime when, with the lifting of wartime constraints, arguments were likely to ensue over property rights in research, if precautions were not taken. The basic principle was that no company should have the exclusive right to exploit patents on research publicly funded by the taxpayer. Thus, licenses were to be made available to all interested parties on the premise that profits from publicly funded research should not accrue to a single company. It was also expected that by licensing more than one company to practice a given invention, competitive forces would keep prices "reasonable."

The issue of university-generated intellectual property arose at the outset of government funding of military research at the universities during World War II. Clearly, such research would produce useful results beyond immediate wartime needs, and these intellectual property rights should be protected. However, there was no decision at the time—nor was such a decision necessary, given the immediate focus on developing technology to win the war—on how those rights should eventually be used. When the federal government continued to fund university research after the war, the issue of disposition of intellectual property rights was not yet clarified.

The Postwar Intellectual Property Regime

The Department of Commerce's National Technical and Information Service (NTIS) centrally managed licensing in the early postwar period. Academic technology is typically embryonic, requiring the active involvement of the inventor for its further development. With the inventor located in the university, but the NTIS controlling the licensing rights, there was a gap between university, government, and industry. Nevertheless, even though the NTIS was physically distant from the source of discoveries, the arrangement worked reasonably well as companies learned about relevant research and approached the government for licenses in fields such as mechanical devices, electronics, and chemical processes, where development costs and product development times—and consequently risks—were low.

By the late 1960s, however, there was increasing evidence of industry's failing to take advantage of many of the results of academic research, paradoxically because these results were "freely available to all." The approach completely broke down in areas with long development timeframes and high costs, such as the pharmaceutical industry. In 1968, a study by the Johnson administration found that no pharmaceutical to which the government owned the patent had ever been developed for commercial use. Companies were unwilling to make the investment required to develop a drug, a cost that could run into many millions of dollars (even before passage of the Food, Drug and Cosmetic Act of 1973 substantially raised the cost of obtaining marketing approval for a new drug), without the guarantee that they would be able to recoup their investment through exclusive marketing rights.

Government was divided internally during the 1970s, with agencies holding various positions on the best course to follow with respect to the intellectual property they had helped create. For example, the Atomic Energy Commission wished to keep title within government to inventions in its domain. Other agencies, such as the National Institutes of Health (NIH) and National Science Foundation, were more willing to assign inventions to sources outside government to facilitate development. Government authorized institutional patent agreements (IPAs) in response to the Johnson administration's study. The Department of Health, Education and Welfare was the first to implement IPAs, followed by the National Science Foundation.

Norman Latker, NIH patent counsel, invented a bureaucratic process for universities to certify that they were taking appropriate measures to manage technology transfer. He developed forms for university administrators to fill out to create a record of their compliance, ideally by establishing professional in-house offices for patenting and licensing (Latker 1998). For universities not wishing to make such an extensive commitment, procedures were created for individual patenting. Because the process could take as long as three years, a school might find that the potential licensee's interest had lapsed by the time the agreement was in place. Moreover, the period of exclusivity under IPAs was restricted to ten years.

Some government officials, in both the legislative and executive branches, strongly believed that these rights were public property and should not be turned over to the universities to be licensed to industry. There was significant opposition in Congress, for example, from Senator Long of Louisiana, who believed that patenting of government-funded research was illegitimate privatization of what should be a free public good. As long as the few interested universities were able to work out ways of accessing rights to the inventions they were interested in commercializing, this issue lay dormant. But when Joseph Califano, secretary of Health, Education and Welfare, called a halt to the transfer of NIH patent rights to universities in the late 1970s and fired its patent counsel, Norman Latker, the issue of what to do with the federal government's growing patent portfolio came to a head (Latker 1998).

The Bayh-Dole Act arose from a debate between opponents and proponents of patenting of government-funded research. Opponents held that research paid for by government should be made freely available to all interested parties. Proponents argued that potentially interested firms would be unlikely to take up this research unless they could be assured of the limited monopoly protection offered by a patent and, preferably, by an exclusive license. The Senate Judiciary Committee found that in 1978, the government owned title to more than twenty-eight thousand patents but had licensed fewer than 4 percent of them (Etzkowitz and Stevens 1995). The virtually unanimous vote in favor of Bayh-Dole resulted in part from the need to respond to the challenge to U.S. industrial competitiveness during the 1970s (Stevens 2004). Because direct programs of government aid to industry were too controversial, an indirect industrial policy, going through the university to reach industry, was instituted.

The Bayh-Dole Regime

The Bayh-Dole Act resolved the contradiction between government's ownership of intellectual property rights in the research that it funded at universities and the wish to see those rights put to use. Bayh-Dole created an intellectual property development system that combined private and public benefits in a balanced framework. It took into account the need to incentivize all participants to advance commercialization and maximize access to the knowledge created with government funds, at one and the same time. While university technology transfer predates Bayh-Dole and was on an upward trajectory at the time of its passage, the act codified and legitimized a set of informal practices and relationships that had emerged among university, industry, and government during the preceding century.

Until recently, relatively few universities maintained an office for taking out and licensing patents. A 1940 survey of sixteen universities reported 380 patents taken out, of which 114 were in active use; the study also found that "only five educational institutions report income from patents" (Potter 1940, 6). Following a gradual increase in the early postwar period, university-held patents rose nearly tenfold between 1979 and 1997, "from 264 to 2,436, as compared with a two-fold increase in the overall number of patents during that period" (Rai and Eisenberg 2003). Was this rise caused by Bayh-Dole, or was it in the making prior to passage of the act and would have occurred anyway, without government intervention (Mowery et al. 2004)? The law of 1980 created a regulatory framework, a new criterion of academic distinction, and revised academia's incentives. New classes of universities entered seriously onto the technology transfer scene after 1980: (1) high-status research universities, such as Columbia, whose previous external orientation had primarily been toward government rather than industry, and (2) rising schools such as Arizona State University, seeking to make a name for themselves as an "entrepreneurial university."

Commitment of resources, internally or from government, and leadership, such as that provided by President Michael Crow of Arizona State, or at least encouragement from university administration, are crucial to success of the project. The turnaround at the Johns Hopkins University in recent years, from disinterest in technology transfer to becoming a model for emulation, exemplifies the importance of a supportive academic environment. A comparative analysis of national experiences suggests that introduction of a Bayh-Dole–like legal regime without concomitant development of the capacity to promote technology transfer is insufficient—as in, for example, the experience of Denmark.[5] By contrast, in Japan, a change in law accompanied by strong government support for development of university technology transfer offices has led to an exponential increase in patenting (Leydesdorff and Meyer, in press).

Bayh-Dole as Indirect Industrial Policy

The Bayh-Dole Act altered the regulatory infrastructure that determined how the results of federally funded research, which would have been funded by government anyway, could be used. Although no funds were appropriated for implementation, universities were able to charge some of the costs of their patent-licensing offices to their administrative overhead rates for federal grants, thus receiving an indirect subsidy. More important initially was the need to meet the requirement of putting research to use to remain eligible for federal funding of research. By this change in the rules of the game—placing responsibility for technology transfer in the university where it was being conducted rather than with government (the funder)—potentially useful research was moved closer to users. In the context of federal research budgets that were not growing at a fast enough rate to meet academic researchers' needs, universities were given the opportunity to earn monies from the royalties and equity they could generate from federally sponsored research on their campuses.

Indirect industrial policy was more fruitful than many more direct schemes. It was not intervention in the sense of specific government measures requiring targeting of particular areas of research and development for support, as occurs in Japan, or requiring enterprises and research institutes to make research contracts with each other, as in the Eastern European socialist model. Instead, incentives were built into the research funding system to move the universities closer to industry in their motivation and structure. This occurred in a context in which government was unable to take more direct measures.

Technology transfer offices view the Bayh-Dole Act as the charter document of their profession. Indeed, some have analogized it as the Magna Carta of academic technology transfer (Etzkowitz and Goktepe 2005). The act provided the impetus for virtually all research universities to become involved in technology transfer, beyond the few that, early on, had identified it as a significant task. The act resolved the free-rider problems that companies faced in dealing with government-owned, university-originated intellectual property. A firm feared that if it went ahead and spent considerable sums to develop a successful technology, a second firm might come along and demand access on the grounds that the technology was funded with taxpayer money. By placing this intellectual property securely within the university, a firm could be guaranteed that when an exclusive license was granted, it would hold.

Technology transfer offices uniformly accept the validity and necessity of the law. It not only provides a basis for technology transfer but also encourages faculty to participate, because they are guaranteed a significant share of income—in contrast to corporate employees, who are at the mercy of their employer.

Moreover, the act opens the way to creation of a new funding stream for academia from the proceeds of technology transfer. Some universities have extended the scope of the Bayh-Dole regime through internal rule-making and claim rights over all intellectual property resulting from university research, on the grounds that the intellectual and social atmosphere of the campus is an essential ingredient to faculty invention. Bayh-Dole and technology transfer offices improve efficiency in the technology transfer process by clarifying individual and organizational roles and by providing guidelines for the sharing of financial rewards. In the decades since passage of the act, the technology transfer office has become an integral part of the university structure. Bayh-Dole gives the university the ability to develop further business capacities that may then allow it to participate in entrepreneurial activities such as venture capital and firm-formation.

Technology transfer offices view themselves as part of the service mission of the university to provide public benefits by putting research to use. Even as the business arm of the university, transfer offices view themselves as promoting core academic values such as dissemination of knowledge through publication and expansion of research (Hatakenaka 2004). They advise on management of conflict-of-interest issues and general university policy on technology transfer. Earning money is important, especially to reach the break-even point of earning enough to pay for the costs of the office and justify its efficacy to the administration, but it is by no means the only objective.[6] The balance between financial and other objectives was exemplified by the decision at Stanford not to integrate the technology transfer office with the university's endowment-management organization, a unit highly oriented to financial maximizations (Sondelin 2004).

Financial goals rarely predominate; most technology transfer offices see their role as providing a range of services for assisting their clients and view profit maximization from technology transfer as one objective to be balanced against assisting academics to put their technology to use, even when the financial rewards are not large. As one technology transfer officer said in reply to a query about return on investment (ROI), "Financial ROI is only one aspect [and often not stronger than other key aspects] that drives most academic institutions' tech transfer offices" (Techno-L Listserve, Jan. 14, 2005). As technology transfer offices secure their financial base, they are more easily able to operate according to a long-range timeframe and to undertake projects that do not have immediate marketability.

Some universities have extended their efforts from the taking out and licensing of patents to produce income for the university to a portfolio of measures designed to establish new firms and thereby promote regional economic development. All of these efforts depend on research staff and students bringing their commercializable ideas to the attention of a university technology transfer office. In part because taking out patents is expensive, universities tend to patent only when a prospective licensee can be identified in advance, an approach originated by Neils Reimers (1992), director of technology licensing at Stanford in the 1970s, and then adopted by MIT and other schools. Most universities patent their intellectual property only when they can be reasonably assured of finding a market for it, although this is changing as longer-range strategies are adopted.

A Virtual "Land Grant"

The Morrill Act of 1862 donated federal land to support the development of higher education for the improvement of agricultural and industrial practice. The Bayh-Dole Act turned over intangible property in scientific and technological knowledge to the universities, with similar intentions. This legislation encouraged individual academics to include commercial activities among their roles and universities to experiment with a variety of arrangements such as research parks, "incubator" facilities, and offices for the transfer of technology to develop fruitful relationships with industry.

Occasionally, a faculty member at a university new to technology transfer manages to circumvent the office and deal directly with the university's patent attorneys, running up a legal bill for an invention without prior assessment of its potential (Marburger 1995). However, every technology transfer officer is on the lookout for a "big fish" and is keenly aware of the need to educate faculty to discern the economic potential of their research. Indeed, the impetus to establish an intellectual property regime has often been the cautionary story of "the one that got away," either because the inventor was unaware of its potential or because the university had not yet established a technology transfer office.

The Bayh-Dole Act provided a stable ground for university technology transfer and a framework for resolving some issues. Of course, other issues remained. The potentially contentious matter of division of proceeds seems to have been settled within the context of Bayh-Dole. The act guarantees the inventor a share through a more or less equal three-way division of proceeds among the university administration on behalf of the institution as a whole, the faculty member's department, and the individual inventor. Student-generated rights were traditionally left entirely with the individual, perhaps on the grounds that students paid tuition and did not have employee status. However, because most graduate students in the sciences are on fellowships, often from a government or university source, graduate students have increasingly been defined as "officers of the university" subject to the same intellectual property rules as faculty.

Whatever the administrative definition, however, student status is different, in reality, from faculty status. Student work is typically conducted under the control of faculty members, and unless a university has clear rules and procedures, whether students are included in disclosure statements can become a matter of faculty discretion. Acknowledgment, both intellectual and pecuniary, of graduate students' research contribution to patents is a below-the-surface issue that rarely comes to light, given faculty members' near feudal power over students in assessing progress toward the Ph.D. and in granting degrees. The academic system has more or less accepted a system of authorship by status, in which provision of resources to conduct research carries with in an entitlement to credit of all kinds. As intellectual property rights become increasingly salient, we can expect that relationships among teachers, students, and the university will have to be more clearly defined.

Access by academic researchers to patented discoveries has also become an issue. In a previous era, when there was a clear distinction between basic and applied research, this was not a great problem, because patenting largely took place away from the research frontier. However, at present, basic discoveries in molecular biology produce practical results simultaneously with research advances, and the issue of access comes to the fore. Bayh-Dole places control over this problem in the hands of the university. Universities can protect access for academic researchers by including provisions in licensing agreements that authorize access.

In the early 1980s, most universities merely hoped to earn enough to pay for the running of a technology transfer office, so that they could satisfy the new government requirement for the university to play a role in support of industry in exchange for receiving government research funds. That level of income was achieved relatively quickly at many universities, almost to their own surprise. Between 2003 and 2005, U.S. universities that took part in the Association of University Technology Managers licensing survey (2005) reported about $1.6 billion in licensing incomes. (Although we should note that a few large returns came from awards in infringement proceedings, in which a company was found to be using patented research without authorization, and from the sale of equity in firms founded with university intellectual property.)

Some observers project an impending "shake-out" of university patent offices that are unable to cover their costs (Sampat and Mowery 2001). This prediction is partly based on a misplaced analogy with the rise and relative decline of the Research Corporation as a major actor on the university intellectual property scene. The shift of RC from a focus on patenting to venture capital was spurred by the decentralization of patent offices across the academic research system. Even at a less intensive level, academic technology transfer efforts have been found to be economically successful. Many observers were skeptical a decade ago, and some still are, that universities could even make enough money from their technology transfer efforts to cover costs (Mowery et al. 2004). The rule is that it takes approximately seven years to reach the break-even point.[7]

The university's own economic base also begins to change as it generates some of its income from the sale of inventions. In 1992, Columbia University earned $24 million from its intellectual property rights, the equivalent of the income on almost half a billion dollars of endowment. This income rose to $100 million by the end of the 1990s, most of it derived from a single patent on the transgenic mouse—a patent that would soon expire. In recognition of this eventuality, the university is expanding its efforts into additional areas such as software. Academic institutions have also begun to use funds earned from technology transfer start-ups to support the operation of the university. Columbia began a $2 million program to support new research initiatives, drawing on monies earned from patents licensed to companies.

The broader underlying process here is the movement of universities away from being eleemosynary, or charitable, institutions that gain their support from other sectors of society. We can predict that they will generate even higher levels of their own support from their research activities, on the assumption that only a small proportion of the academic capacity for translating knowledge into the economy is currently being used. The new arrangements open the possibility that universities will become, at least in part, financially self-supporting institutions—entities obtaining revenues through licensing agreements and other financial arrangements for the industrial use of new knowledge discovered on their campuses.

Controversy over the Economic Consequences of Bayh-Dole

The potential contribution of academia to regional and national economic growth transcends the financial health of academia. The Federal Reserve Bank of Boston produced the classic study of a single institution, estimating that MIT alumni were responsible for founding 4,000 firms that, in 1994 alone, employed at least 1.1 million people and generated $232 billion in world sales (Bank of Boston 1997). This study included effects preceding the Bayh-Dole era and reminds us that the act expanded a phenomenon that was already in motion. A more recent Biotechnology Industry Association–sponsored study, projecting more conservatively from royalty income derived from U.S. university technology transfer, estimated the creation of 279,000 jobs, nationwide, during a twelve-year period (Roessner 2009). While these studies vary in their units of analysis and time periods, they do show significant economic outcomes from academia that go well beyond traditional measures of student spending and research spending.

Patenting, licensing, and firm-formation are three phases of a new academic business model in which intellectual property is created, translated into products, and marketed. The initial two-phase model, relating to existing firms, of course, continues. Moreover, the two models overlap, as an established firm may acquire the start-up once it has demonstrated that academic intellectual property is translatable into a viable product. In 2005 alone, 527 new products were introduced onto the market, and in the eight years from 1998 through 2005, 3,641 new products based on academic inventions were introduced—an average of 1.25 per day. In addition, 628 new spin-offs were created in 2005 (for a total of 5,171 since enactment of Bayh-Dole).

Are universities generating less patentable research in recent years, acting more selectively in choosing what they patent, or becoming shortsighted in not patenting without a customer in hand? In 2004, the invention disclosures among U.S. institutions increased to 16,871, up 8.8 percent from FY 2003, while patents issued decreased 6.4 percent to 3,680. Leydesdorff and Meyer (in press) interpret the recent modest decline in the United States as evidence that universities are reemphasizing the traditional roles measured by highly publicized newspaper surveys. But Sine, Shane, and Di Gregorio

(2003) found that after controlling for other factors, a one-unit increase in an institution's *U.S. News and World Report* ranking increased the rate of licensing by 1.5 percent. Even the negative conclusions of some academic assessments of university technology transfer demonstrate an awareness of the rise of a significant phenomenon, albeit one whose generalizability is still in question (Bania, Eberts, and Fogarty 1993).

The raw data, however, suggest that universities are becoming engines of economic growth (Feller 1990). From 1998 through 2005, about 3,114 new products were introduced to the marketplace by the institutions surveyed by the Association of University Technology Managers (Bostrom and Tieckelmann 2005). U.S. institutions executed nearly 4,800 new licenses or options in 2004, up 6.1 percent from FY 2003, and more than two-thirds were with newly formed or existing small companies. Moreover, recent initiatives by universities to enhance their capacity for firm-formation indicate that they think they can do better.[8] In 2004 alone, 462 new companies based on academic discovery began operation in North America; 74.5 percent were in the originating institution's home state or province, suggesting that investment in technology transfer capabilities has a salutary effect on the local region, rather than their results spilling over to a more attractive venue. However, another study showed that the local effect was greatest when "personal contact" was important to the transfer and differed by sector: significant for electronics but not for instruments (Bania, Eberts and Fogarty 1993).

The Bayh-Dole Act is more than an amendment to patent law, establishing various classes of ownership rights in academia to intellectual property generated from federally sponsored research. Bayh-Dole is a "virtual land grant act" of the Knowledge Era, assigning the intellectual property rights generated from federally funded research to the universities where it is performed in the expectation of generating future economic and social benefits. After passage of the Morrill Act in 1862, the sale of federal lands provided for development of a new class of universities, oriented to the improvement of agriculture, the nation's major industry at the time; in a unique instance, one-third of the Massachusetts land grant went toward founding MIT, to infuse the nation's first technology region with new ideas (Etzkowitz 2002).

The Relationship of Patents to the Academic Mission

The experience at MIT played a key role in defining the relationship among patents, professors, universities, and firms, which later became institutionalized in the Bayh-Dole Act and the common intellectual property regime now emerging in academia internationally. Industry's view of academia as a source of intellectual property before Bayh-Dole was exemplified in a 1980 survey in which fifty-six firms were asked why they funded research at universities (National Science Board 1982). Multiple answers were possible (table 3.1). The last of the reasons cited—obtaining information, unavailable elsewhere, for solving a specific problem—is a good working definition of a proprietary advantage, and yet in 1980 it was the least common explanation of why companies looked to universities. During the 1980s, industry's view of academia began to shift, initially among pharmaceutical companies and then across a broader range of industries interested in discontinuous innovation. Industry began to see academic research as a source of valuable inventions (and patents), to which it needed direct access. The relationship of the pharmaceutical industry to biotechnology firms emerging from universities over the past three decades has been a watershed event that is spreading to other fields such as computational chemistry and nanotechnology.

Patents are a compromise between treating technological knowledge as a "gift" and treating it as a strictly pecuniary asset. The limit of a U.S. patent to twenty years (in contrast to ninety-six years for a copyright), requirements to "use it or lose it," difficulties in enforcement, and provisions for free access for academic researchers—all ensure that the two opposing positions are not an absolute dichotomy.[9] Patents are a "co-opetitive" knowledge format (i.e., one that combines cooperation with competition), integrating free access and privatization. Because patents both publicize and protect intellectual property, they do not pose a threat to dissemination of scientific research findings. Rather, it is the failure to patent that inhibits the broadest dissemination of useful knowledge, by excluding it from the patent database.[10]

The private right conferred by a patent to exclude others from using an invention except through agreement with the originator/owner, usually for monetary consideration, further serves the public interest through the capitalization of knowledge. By allowing an inventor a temporary monopoly, patenting encourages investment in technological innovations and contributes to economic development, because it reduces the risk that others will take free advantage; conversely, lack of such assurance discourages initial investment. This advantage of the patent system has been illustrated in recent years by biotechnology firms, which have been able to obtain long-term investments in part due to their secure patent rights, and by software firms, where patenting is not the norm and firms have had to rely on short-term capital.

TABLE 3.1.
Reasons Cited by Industry for Sponsoring Academic Research,
Survey of 56 Firms, 1980

Reason	Percentage of firms
Gain access to manpower	75
Gain window on science and technology	52
Provide general support for technical excellence	38
Gain access to university facilities	36
Obtain prestige; enhance company's image	32
Act as good local citizen; foster community relations	29
Make use of an economical resource	14
Solve problem; get specific information unavailable elsewhere	11

Source: Data from National Science Board 1982.

The Patent System as "Quasi-University"

Patents are both an information system and a disclosure process, because the invention and its means of achievement become publicly available on issuance. In this sense, the U.S. patent system functions as a "quasi-university," collating, validating, and disseminating technologies and knowledge about technology. The "patent university" has long functioned without face-to-face communication, while the "bricks-and-mortar" university is just now beginning to explore the potential of the "virtual" university by developing distance-learning capabilities.

The founders of the modern patent system created a knowledge network in the early nineteenth century, linking dispersed inventors to one another through a central node that qualified, certified, and dispensed information.[11] Dissemination was made more efficient by providing a decentralized storage and dissemination system, using libraries as a distribution mechanism in an era of relatively poor communication. Moreover, the patent system raised the level of the knowledge disseminated by subjecting it to a critical analytical and winnowing process through a system of patent examiners and by setting criteria for novelty and utility.

Through its licensing fees, the patent system also provided an incentive to inventors to share their knowledge. This financial incentive is typically noted as an aspect of early U.S. industrial policy, because it created an organizational mechanism for government intervention in the economy. But the patent system was more than industrial policy. In an era before today's almost universal higher education, and in parallel with the rise of the land-grant university, the patent system functioned as a "distributed technological university." Clearly, the patent system is like a university in only some ways, such as that it distributes knowledge and functions as a collective means of generating new knowledge.

The U.S. patent system, then, served as an early distance-learning university and invisible research group, comprising the inventors working on a particular topic who read and cited one another's patents. In contrast to the United Kingdom, where patent fees were high and access to the patent system was limited, the U.S. patent system encouraged broad access through a minimal fee structure and made technical knowledge available at low cost through the postal system and large public libraries designated as patent depository libraries (Dobyns 1994).

Patents were organized by categories, with sorting mechanisms, long before relational databases in software became available. To this day, through the internet and CD-ROMs, inventors use the patent system for research and educational purposes. Further invention is thus encouraged by learning about gaps in technology and about advances that can be further extended or worked around. The classic instance of this serial invention modality is the inventor of xerography, Chester Carlson, whose "daytime job" was as a patent attorney. Carlson studied the patent literature to identify gaps in copying technology and hints of how processes could be improved, by working within the lacunae and from the achievements of the cohort of inventors in this field—exemplifying the relationship between the individual and collective nature of invention.

Patents facilitate the innovation process by creating a social framework for technological advance. Organized in online databases, the collectivity of patents provides an inspiration to inventors seeking innovation. Entrepreneurial scientists and their research groups, as well as existing firms searching for new ideas, find their way to each other. The Bayh-Dole regime provides a mechanism for these interests to meet and to be mediated by universities' technology transfer offices, in a way that adds value to an invention and reduces friction in transfer.

Economic and social development increasingly originates in academia as protected intellectual property, with the university assisted by government— through regulatory and venture capital initiatives—to become the source of future industry as well as new knowledge. The university is taking an entrepreneurial role formerly played by industry, alone or with government, and is the source of new firms. Universities themselves are taking additional steps to assist faculty and students to develop the commercial as well as intellectual implications of their research, offering access to financing and business assistance to form a firm. The seed venture capital function is being internalized within the university following the path of intellectual property protection.

Conclusion

As the university contributes to economic and social development, it is empowered to protect its interests. Fear of industry dominance of universities is superseded by firms' concern that a university-originated start-up may displace them. The transition from the teaching to the research university provided a template for managing conflicts, such as the one-fifth rule regulating consultation; it was also the first step toward the entrepreneurial academic transition, followed by contracts with large firms and encouragement of start-ups. While overlapping roles generate conflicts of interest, they also produce useful confluences. The technology transfer office provides an administrative mechanism to negotiate the academic-industrial interface and manage conflicts, protecting publication and dissemination while simultaneously capturing profit and encouraging enterprise and regional development.

A relatively common entrepreneurial mode is emerging in academic systems with diverse traditions and norms (Etzkowitz et al. 2008). Lacking a technology transfer interface, the Swedish "professors' exemption"—deriving from medieval precedent exempting academics from ordinary citizens' obligations, such as quartering soldiers in their homes—had the unintended consequence of limiting commercialization of research to the activities of a relatively small number of highly entrepreneurially oriented faculty members (Goktepe 2008). In effect, the U.S. Bayh-Dole Act created a "partial professors' exemption" by guaranteeing academic inventors a significant share of pecuniary rewards, while encouraging the creation of technology transfer interface mechanisms to sort ownership claims among putative inventors and provide services to the middle range of faculty who want their research commercialized but do not wish to take the lead themselves. Nevertheless, the Swedish and U.S. models are convergent in, on the one hand, carving out individual inventors' rights from the interests of their employers and, on the other hand, inserting a commercialization support structure within and around the university, such as the government-funded Technology Bridge Foundations in Sweden and venture capital firms and incubator facilities in the United States. Even as the ostensibly private U.S. model is transferred to

Sweden, the more public Swedish model appears in the United States, through state governments' technology development foundations in the fifty states and various federal programs such as Small Business Innovation Research.

An entrepreneurial university, uniting teaching, research, and commercialization of knowledge, is at the heart of economic development efforts, from Baltimore to Rio de Janeiro, Leuven, and Johannesburg: diverse yet prototypical instances of the shift toward direct involvement by leading academic institutions in enterprise development.

Coevolution is a mutual process of change that reorients the institutional spheres in a common direction. This process may take place through covariation, with two or more spheres introducing organizational innovations to reach a common goal. As the university has taken on some of the traditional role of business, government has revised the patent system. As the university has internalized the capabilities to patent, the patent system has moved toward allowing patenting of discoveries nearer the "basic" end of the spectrum.

This development reflects a change in the nature of knowledge itself, a shift from dual formats such as "applied" and "basic" to a unitary model of "polyvalent knowledge" exhibiting multiple characteristics simultaneously (Viale and Etzkowitz 2004). The useful potential of knowledge is moving from the so-called Edison's Quadrant of special focus on useful knowledge to Pasteur's dual focus and into Bohr's Quadrant of knowledge for its own sake, as well (Stokes 1999). Indeed, the notion of separate quadrants is reaching "technological obsolescence" as "basic" knowledge increasingly exhibits practical implications, and vice versa—the movement toward knowledge produced in the context of application has its counterpart in applications produced in the context of basic research (Gibbons et al. 1994).

This is also the fundamental reason that other countries, from Sweden to Italy and Brazil, are attempting to find their own ways to use the patent system to foster knowledge-based economic development from their academic institutions. Sweden has established university "holding companies" to purchase intellectual property rights from their owners, who according to Sweden's 1949 academic law are the individual professors. In Italy, a new law grants such rights to the professor, thus clarifying an unclear legal situation that encouraged paralysis and left room for only limited informal transfer of rights and their use (Viale 2001). The Bayh-Dole regime, with its provisions for transparency and sharing between the academic institution and the actual inventors (faculty, students, and staff), is an ideal toward which many countries currently strive.

The patent system plays a significant supporting role in the transition from the research to the entrepreneurial university. As efforts to commercialize academic research get under way in Europe and Japan, offers to pay for taking out a patent in exchange for part of the rights have resulted in a division between the university and the individual professor. Under these conditions, case-by-case negotiations are soon superseded by precedent as the basis for a division of proceeds between the individual, the research unit or department, and the university. As precedent takes hold, a one-third rule is elaborated internationally, whether by law, as in Denmark, or through purchase of a share of the rights, as in Sweden (Norman 2005). The relatively autonomous position of the professor in the university, in comparison to the scientist as employee of a corporation, is the fundamental basis for this shared intellectual property regime. Whether speeded by law or developed more slowly through precedent, the outcome is basically the same; so are the issues that must be resolved.

Initially, as with research in the late nineteenth century, the new academic mission is defined as a conflict of interest with the old. Over time, new legitimating themes are identified to make the opposing themes compatible (e.g., "research enhances teaching, and vice versa"). Confluences of interest, such as "the economic development mission supports the research mission of the university," are discovered. Moreover, legal changes such as the Bayh-Dole Act, legitimizing an academic patenting regime, or the 1998 amendment to the constitution of the State of Oklahoma, allowing public universities to accept stock in companies as payment for intellectual property developed on campus, accelerate the process of organizational and normative change.

Conflict-of-interest issues are the subject of increasingly sophisticated policies that create a balance between ensuring independence of judgment and putting the most expert knowledge to use in addressing a problem.[12] Going too far in one direction or the other can impede either objective, as the editors of a leading medical journal found when they excluded from the reviewing process anyone with pecuniary interest in the research topic. The editors of the *New England Journal of Medicine* soon found that they could not get knowledgeable reviewers with this criterion in place, and they amended the rule to simply require disclosure of financial interest and excluded only those persons with a direct interest in a firm rather than a field.

Academic patenting and the broader issue of the university's role in economic and social development, as well as older issues of the balance between research and teaching, are a matter of continuing controversy and debate. U.S. academic patenting is an organizational innovation with a unique provenance in academic entrepreneurialism. However, it is but one answer to the question of the academic role in the knowledge economy in an era when the university is a major research producer. Other academic systems, such as in postwar Japan, Italy, and Sweden, transfer commercializable research findings in exchange for research funds and consulting opportunities. Nevertheless, Japan, Germany, and Denmark recently adopted a regulatory structure based on the Bayh-Dole model (Kneller 1999; Krucken 2003). It remains to be seen whether legal changes can lead or must lag the development of organizational capacity for technology transfer and the emergence of an entrepreneurial ethos as drivers of change in the university. In any event, a shift in focus is under way, from an emphasis on licensing to incubation, venture capital, and firm-formation.

In the not too distant past, many schools modeled themselves on Harvard, calling themselves "the Harvard" of their region. Currently, Harvard models itself on MIT, the classical entrepreneurial university. Recently, Harvard alumni returning for their forty-fifth reunion were taken on a bus tour of MIT and its penumbra of biotechnology and pharmaceutical firms. They were told that the surrounding area of their own university was going to look like MIT's in the future, only on a larger scale, as Harvard has greater resources to hire entrepreneurial faculty and encourage spin-offs (J. Marlin, personal communication, Oct. 2007).

The ivory tower university is becoming the entrepreneurial university, even as the Humboldtian framework of academic independence persists as its core. Indeed, the ability of the university to earn money from its intellectual property rights, through the licensing of inventions and receipt of equity in spin-off firms, potentially gives it an enhanced degree of independence as it generates some of its own resources. The boundaries between university, industry, and government shift as academia plays a larger role in economic development. The enhanced role of the university is sometimes hidden by ideological commitments to earlier academic modes that nevertheless remain an essential part of the academic enterprise. The relative influence of actors in increasingly knowledge-based societies shifts toward the one with the most highly valued good. Formerly a secondary, supporting institution, the university becomes coequal with government and industry, the leading institutions in modern society since the eighteenth century.

NOTES

1. "At the time the [Research] Corporation began to stir, the universities were awakening to the predicament into which the new relations between science and industry, or research and commercialization had placed them. Who if anyone should protect the patentable results flowing form academic laboratories? Should not the universities whose facilities produced the results? And ought not educational institutions to prosecute their rights with what vigor they could manage during the downturn in the economy, to offset losses in endowment income and state allocations? But then, would it not be compromising, and even immoral, to obtain royalties from inventions made at tax exempt institutions supported by public monies or private gifts?" (Heilbron and Seidel 1989, 104).

2. Information from a Stanford administrator responsible for the university's office of technology licensing; interview with the author, July 2005.

3. Information from a representative of the Stanford Management Corporation; interview with the author, Aug. 2005.

4. The award was given jointly to Banting and J. J. R. Macleod, the academic sponsor of the research. Banting split his prize money with Best, and Macleod with J. B. Collip, the biochemist on the project. The appropriate allocation of credit became part of the issue of ownership when it was realized that this was necessary to ensure a valid patent.

5. Lissoni et al. (2009) offer, as an alternative interpretation, that cultural and organizational ties of professors and universities to existing firms are so strong that intellectual property rights devolve to them, irrespective of the intellectual property regime.

6. Indeed, at CERN, the multinational-sponsored European Organization for Nuclear Research—a non-university research institute—earnings are beside the point. The objective of the technology transfer office is to demonstrate the utility of particle physics to the larger society, beyond solving fundamental problems of cosmology, typically through contribution to medical imaging technologies (B, Denis, Associate Director, Technology Transfer CERN, personal communication, Sept. 2009).

7. For metrics of economic outcomes of academic patenting, see Etzkowitz and Stevens 1995.

8. For a variety of initiatives, see *Technology Transfer Tactics* 3 (9): 129–44, 2009.

9. For example, the debate over the stem cell patent held by the Wisconsin Alumni Research Foundation resulted in an arrangement negotiated to give universities licenses for a nominal fee. In practice, academic researchers have declared a de facto right to free access. For a discussion of various modalities, within the context of intellectual property rights, to facilitate knowledge flow within and among academia and industry, see Bergman and Graf 2007.

10. See Mowery et al. 2001. The argument that leading universities already involved in patenting would have gone ahead irrespective of Bayh-Dole is undoubtedly correct. Indeed, the data presented here delineate the early provenance of academic patenting in the United States. Nevertheless, the broader impact of the act probably lies in the legitimatization and expansion of the activity to a broader range of universities, transforming the activity from an anomaly into a taken-for-granted enterprise. See the Association of University Technology Managers website (www.autm.net) for additional statistics on academic patenting.

11. Authority to grant patents was included in the Constitution, art. 1, sect. 8, the implicit warrant for U.S. science and technology policy, but a formal organizational mechanism, beyond assignment of responsibility to the secretary of state to implement this intention, was not put in place until 1836.

12. See, for example, Stanford University Research Policy Handbook, Conflict of Commitment and Interest for Academic Staff (http://rph.stanford.edu/4–4.html).

REFERENCES

Apple, R. 1989. Patenting university research: Harry Steenbock and the Wisconsin Alumni Research Foundation. *Isis* 30:375–94.

Association of University Technology Managers. 2000. Licensing survey. www.autm.net.

Bania, N., R. Eberts, and M. Fogarty. 1993. Universities and the startup of new companies: Can we generalize from Silicon Valley and Route 128? *Review of Economics and Statistics* 75 (4): 761–66.

Bank of Boston. 1997. *MIT: The Impact of Innovation*. Boston: Federal Reserve Bank of Boston.

Bechtel, K. 1985. Deviant scientists and deviant behavior. *Deviant Behavior* 6:237–52.

———. 2000 Scientific deviance. In *Encyclopedia of Criminology and Deviant Behavior*, ed. C. Bryant. London: Taylor and Francis.

Bergman, K., and G. Graff. 2007. The global stem cell patent landscape: Implications for efficient technology transfer and commercial development. *Nature Biotechnology* 25:419–24.

Bliss, M. 1982. *The Discovery of Insulin*. Chicago: University of Chicago Press.

Bostrom, D., and R. Tieckelmann. 2005. AUTM U.S. licensing survey, FY 2005 survey summary. www.autm.net.

Bush, V. 1970. *Pieces of the Action*. New York: Morrow.

Cyranowski, D. 2006. Why did Hwang fake his data, how did he get away with it, and how was the fraud found out? *Nature*, Jan. 11. www.nature.com.

Dobyns, K. 1994. *The Patent Office Pony: A History of the Early Patents Offices*. Fredericksburg, VA: Sergeant Kirkland's Press.

Etzkowitz, H. 1996. Conflict of interest and commitment in academic science. *Minerva* 34 (3): 259–77.

———. 2002. *MIT and the Rise of Entrepreneurial Science*. London: Routledge.

———. 2008. *The Triple Helix: University-Industry-Government Innovation in Action*. London: Routledge.

Etzkowitz, H., and D. Goktepe. In press. The co-evolution of the university technology transfer office and the linear model of innovation. *International Journal of Technology Transfer*.

Etzkowitz, H. , M. Ranga, M. Benner, L. Guaranys, A. Maculan, and R. Kneller. 2008. Pathways to the entrepreneurial university: Towards a global convergence. *Science and Public Policy* 35 (9): 681–95.

Etzkowitz, H., and A. Stevens. 1995. Inching toward industrial policy: The university's role in government initiatives to assist small innovative companies in the U.S. *Science Studies* 2 (Dec.): 13–31.

Feller, I. 1990. Universities as engines of R&D-based economic growth: They think they can. *Research Policy* 19 (4): 335–48.

Florence, R. 2007. *Lawrence and Aaronsohn: T. E. Lawrence, Aaron Aaronsohn, and the Seeds of the Arab-Israeli Conflict.* New York: Penguin Group.

Gibbons, M., C. Limogens, H. Nowotny, S. Schwartzman, P. Scott, and M. Trow. 1994. *The New Production of Knowledge.* Beverly Hills, CA: Sage.

Goktepe, D. 2008. *Inside the Ivory Tower: Inventors and Patents at Lund University.* Lund: Lund University Press.

Gustin, B. 1975. The emergence of the German chemical profession, 1790–1867. Ph.D. diss., University of Chicago.

Hatakenaka, S. 2004. *University-Industry Partnerships in MIT, Cambridge, and Tokyo.* London: Routledge.

Heilbron, J. L., and R. Seidel, R. 1989. *Lawrence and His Laboratory: A History of the Lawrence Berkeley Laboratory.* Berkeley: University of California Press.

Jencks, C., and D. Riesman. 1968. *The Academic Revolution.* New York: Doubleday.

Kneller, R. 1999. Intellectual property rights and university-industry transfer in Japan. *Science and Public Policy* 26 (2): 113–24.

Krucken, G. 2003. Learning the "new, new thing": On the role of path dependency in university structures. *Higher Education* 46 (3): 315–39.

Latker, N. 1998. Former patent counsel, National Institutes of Health. Interview with author, July 25.

Lécuyer, C. 1992. The making of a science-based technological university: Karl Compton, James Killian and the reform of MIT, 1930–1957. *History of the Physical and Biological Sciences* 23 (1): 153–80.

Leydesdorff, L., and M. Meyer. In press. The decline of university patenting and the end of the Bayh-Dole effect. *Scientometrics.*

Lissoni, F., P. Lotz, J. Schovsbo, and A. Treccani. 2009 Academic patenting and the professor's privilege: Evidence on Denmark from the KEINS database. *Science and Public Policy* 36 (8): 595–60.

Marburger, J. 1995. Former president, Stony Brook University. Interview with author. Apr.

Merton, R. K. 1938. *Science, Technology, and Society in Seventeenth Century England.* Bruges: St. Catherine Press.

———. 1973 [1942]. The normative structure of science. In *The Sociology of Science.* Chicago: University of Chicago Press.

MIT. 1932. Institute policy regarding patents. Massachusetts Institute of Technology Archives, collection AC 64, box 2, folder 3.

———. 1936. Statement concerning patent policy for the 1936 Annual Meeting of the Corporation, dated Oct. 14. Massachusetts Institute of Technology Archives, collection AC 4, box 2, folder 3.

Mowery, D., R. Nelson, B. Sampat, and A. Ziedonis. 2001. The growth of patenting and licensing by U.S. universities: An assessment of the Bayh-Dole Act of 1980. *Research Policy* 30:99–119.

———. 2004. *Ivory Tower and Industrial Innovation.* Stanford, CA: Stanford University Press.

National Science Board. 1982. *University-Industry Relations.* Washington, DC: National Science Foundation.

Norman, C. 2005. Publicly funded support of technology-based ventures. Linkoping studies in science and technology. Thesis no. 1219, Department of Management and Economics, Linkoping University, Sweden.

Potter, A. A. 1940. Research and invention in engineering colleges. *Science* 91 (2349): 6.

Pupin, M. 1923. *From Immigrant to Inventor.* New York: Scribner's.

Rai, A. K., and R. S. Eisenberg. 2003. Bayh-Dole reform and the progress of biomedicine. *Law and Contemporary Problems* 66 (Spring): 289–314.

Reimers, N. 1992. Former director of technology licensing, Stanford University. Interview with author.

Roessner, D. 2009. *The Economic Impact of Licensed Commercialized Inventions Originating in University Research, 1996–2007.* Washington DC: Biotechnology Industry Association. www.bio.org/ip/techtransfer.

Sampat, B., and D. Mowery. 2001. Patenting and licensing university: Lessons from the history of the Research Corporation. *Industrial and Corporate Change* 10 (2): 317–55.

Schmidt, P. 2001. States push public universities to commercialize research. *Chronicle of Higher Education*, Mar. 29: A26–27.

Shapiro, S. 2002. *Tangled Loyalties: Conflict of Interest in Legal Practice.* Ann Arbor: University of Michigan.

Slaughter, S., and G. Rhodes. 2004. *Academic Capitalism and the New Economy.* Baltimore: Johns Hopkins University Press

Sine, W., S. Shane, and D. Di Gregorio. 2003. The halo effect and technology licensing: The influence of institutional prestige on the licensing of university inventions management. *Science* 49 (4): 478–96.

Sondelin, J. 2004. Office of Technology Licensing, Stanford University. Interview with author. Oct.

Stevens, A. 2004. The enactment of Bayh-Dole. *Journal of Technology Transfer* 29:93–99.

Stokes, D. 1999. *Pasteur's Quadrant.* Washington, DC: Brookings Institute.

Viale, R. 2001. Ricerca e innovazione e Stati Uniti. www.farmindustria,.it/scienza2.pdf.

Viale, R., and H. Etzkowitz. 2004. The third academic revolution: Polyvalent knowledge: The DNA of the triple helix. Theme paper presented at Triple Helix V Conference. www.triplehelix5.com.

Washburn, J. 2005. *University Inc. The Corporate Corruption of Higher Education.* New York: Basic Books

CHAPTER 4

Ties That Bind

Relationships among Academia, Industry, and Government in Life Sciences Research

ERIC G. CAMPBELL, PH.D., DARREN E. ZINNER, PH.D.,
GREG KOSKI, PH.D., M.D., AND
DAVID BLUMENTHAL, M.D., M.P.P.

The life sciences enterprise has changed dramatically in the past fifty years. At one time, the domains of academia, industry, and government existed largely as parallel universes. Scientific discoveries from the universities were applied and developed independently by industry to create marketable products and thereby build shareholder equity under the watchful eye of government regulators. This separation no longer exists.

Today, we find the roles and interests of universities, corporations, and government intimately intertwined in a complex combination of financial, intellectual, personal, and legal relationships. On the one hand, these relationships seem to have fostered collaboration, productivity, innovation, and wealth. On the other hand, many observers find them troubling because the competing commitments and interests that result may threaten the integrity of the scientific endeavor itself, particularly in the biomedical and health-related sciences.

In this chapter, we present data regarding the nature, extent, and consequences of the "triple helix" of relationships among academia, government, and industry in the life and health-related sciences.

The Structure of Relationships

For the purpose of this chapter, relationships with industry are defined as arrangements in which academic or government scientists or administrators carry out research or provide intellectual property in return for considerations of various types (research support, honoraria, consulting fees, royalties, equity, etc.). The following types of relationships are among the most common, but this is not an exhaustive listing.

Research relationships: support by industry, usually through a grant or contract, of university-based research (Blumenthal, Campbell, et al. 1996).

Consulting relationships: compensated provision of advice or information, usually by an individual academic or government scientist or administrator, to commercial organizations. Examples of consulting relationships include, but are not limited to, service on boards of directors, service on scientific advisory boards, and so forth (Jones 2000).

Licensing relationships: licensing of government- or university-owned technologies to industry. These relationships are often negotiated and managed by an office of technology transfer located within the government, university, or medical school, and often within independent hospitals and research facilities (Kauffman Foundation Scientific Advisory Committee 2003).

Equity relationships: participation by academic or government scientists in the founding and/or ownership of new companies commercializing university- or government-based research. Equity relationships can stem from consulting and licensing relationships, described above. For example, relationships of this type often occur when cash-poor start-up companies use equity to compensate faculty for consulting or other services in lieu of cash payments. However, scientists may also participate in the founding of new commercial entities, sometimes taking much larger amounts of equity in return for contributions of intellectual property (Bowie 1994).

Training relationships: support by individual companies for the research or educational expenses of graduate students or postdoctoral fellows, or contracts with academic institutions to provide various educational experiences (such as seminars or fellowships) to industrial employees (Blumenthal, Causino, et al. 1996).

Gift relationships: transfers of scientific and nonscientific resources, independent of an institutionally negotiated research grant or contract, from industry to academic or government scientists. Examples of gifts include, but are not limited to, funds for discretionary spending, equipment, food, trips to meetings, biomaterials, and so forth (Campbell, Blumenthal, and Louis 1998).

Institutional relationships: creation of super-relationships with individual companies that support several academic research groups, particularly in interdisciplinary fields. These relationships also exist when the university owns equity in start-up firms that were spun off from academic technology transfer activities (Campbell et al. 2004).

These and other forms of relationship may occur singly or in combination. Combinations of relationships—involving, for instance, research support, gifts, and consulting fees—often raise the most troubling conflict-of-interest concerns, because multiple relationships often involve more money (both real and potential).

The Prevalence and Magnitude of Relationships
Academic-Industry Relationships

While the size of the research and development enterprise within universities is growing, the proportion of it that is funded by industry has remained essentially flat since the early 1980s. Survey data of select institutions by the National Science Foundation, Division of Science Resources Statistics (2004), suggest that roughly two-thirds of all academic research and development is funded by federal and state grants, while only 6 to 7 percent is funded by industrial sources. Yet funding is only one way that academic-industry relationships (AIRs) are created: since passage of the Bayh-Dole Act in 1980, universities have been increasing their efforts to commercialize the results of their research, regardless of the original funding source. Thus, the number of AIRs has grown considerably.

Relationships are particularly prevalent in the life sciences because, compared with other industries, life sciences corporations are much more interested in university research. In a survey by Carnegie Mellon, 58 percent of respondents from pharmaceutical firms reported using public research as a source for new project ideas, compared with an average of 32 percent for the other industries (Cohen, Nelson, and Walsh 2002). When listing the academic-industry channels that are "moderately" or "very" important, pharmaceutical firms, compared with the entire sample of thirty-four industries, placed greater emphasis on academic patenting (50.0% vs. 17.5%), academic licensing (33.8% vs. 9.5%), contract research (52.9% vs. 20.9%), consulting (58.8% vs. 31.8%), and personnel exchange (8.8% vs. 5.8%).

The most recent nationally representative data on the prevalence and magnitude of AIRs in the life sciences stem from surveys of company executives and faculty members conducted in the mid-1990s. A 1994 survey of senior executives of science companies revealed that more than 90 percent of the firms responding to the survey participated in some form of academic-industry relationship. The most prevalent form was retention of university faculty as consultants (88%). Fifty-nine percent of the firms supported university-based research in the form of a grant or contract, and 38 percent supported the training of students and postdoctoral fellows. Seven percent of the firms reported that faculty members were significant equity holders in their companies (Blumenthal, Causino, et al. 1996).

In a 1995 survey of 2,052 faculty members at the fifty most research-intensive U.S. universities, 28 percent of respondents reported receiving some research support from industrial sources (Blumenthal, Campbell, et al. 1996). The prevalence of support was greater for researchers in clinical departments (36%) than those in nonclinical departments (21%). This finding is probably explained by the fact that clinical trials and other forms of clinical research are conducted in clinical departments rather than in basic science departments.

Another recurrent form of relationship was based on consulting. Among basic scientists at the fifty most research-intensive universities in the United States, 60 percent had consulted in the three preceding years (35.2% for a private company and 24.5% for a public company). Among the 60 percent that consulted, 26 percent reported these activities as a major source of supplementary income (Jones 2000).

In the life sciences, academicians frequently serve as principal investigators and sub-investigators for industry-sponsored clinical trials. The nature of the relationship varies, depending on whether the clinical investigation represents a single-site, investigator-originated protocol or a multicenter, sponsor-driven trial. The former is more akin to a sponsored research project, albeit one with a strong interest from the sponsoring firm. In the latter, the physician-investigator often serves as a paid contractor for the sponsoring pharmaceutical firm, recruiting and enrolling study subjects through a standardized protocol. In 2001, the Food and Drug Administration (FDA) recorded more than thirty-eight thousand physicians serving as principal investigators on industry-sponsored protocols. Interestingly, while the absolute number of clinical trial contracts with university medical centers remained essentially stable, academics' share of the total market dropped from nearly

70 percent of trial sites in 1991 to just over one-third in 2001 (Kush et al. 2002). As the clinical trial industry has grown, dedicated research centers and community-based, private practice physicians have begun to conduct trials on behalf of biopharmaceutical sponsors.

The most commonly reported relationship was a gift relationship between academic scientists and industry (Campbell, Blumenthal, and Louis 1998). In our 1998 study, we found that among life sciences faculty in the fifty most research-intensive universities, almost half (43%) received research gifts, independent of a grant or contract from the industry in the three years preceding the study. The most widely reported gifts received from industry were biomaterials (24%), discretionary funds (15%), research equipment (11%), trips to professional meetings (11%), and support for students (9%).

Another source of data regarding scientists' relationships with industry is a review of the University of California, San Francisco (UCSF), annual faculty disclosure forms from 1990 to 1999 (Boyd and Bero 2000). This study found that 7.6 percent of principal investigators at UCSF had some kind of personal financial tie to industry. One-third of the principal investigators reported temporary speaking engagements for companies, one-third held paid positions on scientific advisory boards or boards of directors, and 14 percent reported ownership of equity in a firm. Finally, of the 7.6 percent of principal investigators who reported having financial ties to industry, 12 percent had multiple relationships, including, but not limited to, equity ownership, consulting income, and management interests.

A final source of data on AIRs is a series of case studies examining the extent to which senior leaders of four of the largest, most research-intensive academic health centers in the United States had relationships with industry (Campbell et al. 2004). Examples of study participants included university presidents, provosts or chancellors, medical school deans, vice-deans for research, chairs of life sciences and medical school departments, investment officials, directors of development, directors of technology transfer, directors of public affairs, chief financial officers, development officers, general counsel, and members of institutional review boards (IRBs). In forty-nine confidential interviews across the four institutions, the vast majority of the university officials reported at least one relationship with industry. Examples of officials' relationships included having founded companies, owning equity in companies they had participated in founding, being paid as speakers, and serving as trustees and consultants. Many respondents reported engaging in several of these relationships.

Government-Industry Relationships

The full extent of relationships between scientists at government agencies and corporations is unknown. This does not mean that these government-industry relationships (GIRs) do not exist. Opportunities for such relationships, involving consulting arrangements and equity positions, are certainly not unique to the biomedical and health-related sciences. Without much difficulty, one can imagine a government physicist or engineer entering into such a relationship with a defense or aerospace contractor. Unless the information is disclosed, either through mandatory public financial disclosure or investigative reporting, the public is not likely to know whether or not such relationships do, in fact, occur.

There are no comprehensive, systematically collected, publicly available data that could be used to explore the nature and extent of relationships between government scientists and administrators and industry. Nevertheless, some data came to light in late 2003 and early 2004 with the publication of a series of newspaper articles detailing financial relationships between senior scientists at the National Institutes of Health (NIH) and industry partners, raising significant concern about the nature and extent of these relationships (Willman 2004).

In 1995, the NIH revised its policies for requiring public disclosure of financial statements by highly compensated employees, including senior scientists. The threshold for triggering public disclosure was raised to a level that resulted in a 64 percent decrease in the number of open public disclosures of financial statements. Between 1995 and 2004, consulting relationships between NIH scientists and industry increased, with some accounts estimating that 228 NIH researchers (of 6,000 in all) maintained 365 research agreements from which they collected annual consulting fees in the tens of thousands of dollars and stock options worth as much as $300,000 (Grady 2004). In some cases, these were relationships with companies that stood to benefit financially from the actions of NIH officials. These revelations led the director of the NIH to convene a special advisory group to explore the background and propriety of such relationships (Marshall 2003). This report, and the subsequent congressional hearings on GIRs, led to a strict NIH conflict-of-interest policy, the details of which are provided later in the chapter. Finally, in February 2005, the director of the NIH instituted a moratorium on all relationships between NIH employees and pharmaceutical companies, biotech-

nology companies, trade associations, health care providers, and similar organizations. Although the move was strongly endorsed by the Association of
American Medical Colleges (Cohen 2005), it generated a strong backlash within
the NIH itself. A similar policy has not been instituted at other government
agencies such as the Centers for Disease Control and Prevention or the FDA.

Benefits Associated with Industry Relationships

There is growing empirical evidence that academic-industry relationships
can provide important benefits. Most of the existing literature focuses on the
institutional benefits that accrue as a result of research relationships. However, a small body of evidence has emerged that documents the personal financial benefits that result from consulting relationships.

Funding for University Research

The most obvious benefit of research relationships with industry is that
these arrangements provide funds to support the research conducted in academic institutions. A 1994 survey of senior research executives at 306 life
sciences companies in the United States reported that these companies had
supported more than fifteen hundred academic-based research projects at a
cost of more than $340 million (Blumenthal, Causino, et al. 1996). Based
on these reports, it was estimated that the life sciences industry as a whole
supported more than six thousand projects and expended $1.5 billion on
academic-based research in the life sciences.

Academic Productivity

Contrary to common belief, the receipt of research funding from industry
is not associated with detectable adverse effects on academic productivity. Instead, such research funding is associated with significantly greater academic
productivity on the part of involved university investigators. In our 1994–95
survey of more than two thousand life sciences faculty, those with funding
from industry had published significantly more articles in peer-reviewed journals in the previous three years than faculty without industry funding (14.6
vs. 10.1, respectively; $p < .05$) (Blumenthal, Campbell, et al. 1996). Because
of the cross-sectional nature of the data, we cannot establish causality between industry funding and increased productivity. It may be that industry

funding provides resources that serve to increase investigators' publication productivity. Alternatively, it may be that industry seeks out the most productive researchers. While we cannot know for sure, some combination of these two explanations is most likely at work.

Academic researchers benefit from increased publications, because reports of original research in peer-reviewed journals are one of the main criteria by which faculty are awarded promotions, tenure, prizes, future research grants, positions in professional organizations, and, ultimately, a place in the history of the scientific endeavor (Fox 1985). At an institutional level, a greater number of publications by faculty translates into greater prestige and, perhaps, an increased ability to attract top students, faculty, and future research funding.

Commercial Productivity

In addition to publications, AIRs are associated with an increased likelihood of commercial activities. Faculty with industry funding were significantly more likely than those without such funding to report that they had applied for a patent (42% vs. 24%), had a patent granted (25% vs. 12.6%), had a patent licensed (18.5% vs. 8.7%), had a product under review (26.7% vs. 5.5%), had a product on the market (26.1% vs. 10.8%), or had a start-up company (14.3% vs. 6.0%) (Blumenthal, Campbell, et al. 1996). A number of benefits may accrue to faculty as a result of these commercial opportunities, including financial returns, the opportunity to see the results of their research developed into useful products and services, and, perhaps, enhanced career opportunities in the industrial sector.

Universities also benefit from faculty commercialization. Institutional policies often provide universities with the option to participate in commercial ventures, such as by contributing to the costs of filing a patent in exchange for a portion of the licensing revenues or by providing venture capital funding for a start-up in exchange for a share of its future profits. On rare occasions, universities have also reaped sizable rewards from royalties on licensed patents and from the sale of equity in start-up companies that were based on faculty research.

Early Access to Cutting-Edge Information, Data, and Materials

One of the most important benefits of AIRs for academic researchers and industry alike may be that these relationships allow for the bidirectional flow of the most recent research results. Research relationships with industry often allow a commercial sponsor 30 to 90 days to review the results of the research it sponsored before submission for publication. An executive of a company said that in his field, the published literature is "miles behind the front line of what is happening in universities" (Bowie 1994, 48). For faculty, relationships with industry provide access to industry biomaterials (such as cell lines, reagents, and tissues), equipment, and other research-related resources that may not be available otherwise.

Personal Compensation

There are no comprehensive, publicly available data on the personal financial benefits that accrue to individual scientists or administrators as a result of their relationships with industry. To our knowledge, the only published data stem from the analyses of faculty's annual disclosure forms at UCSF, as described above (Boyd and Bero 2000). Of the 488 faculty disclosures examined, 34 percent were honoraria in the form of occasional speaking fees that produced, on average, $2,500 per year. Of the individuals who received industry money for public speaking, 90 percent received less than $10,000 annually. Consulting arrangements also produced income for UCSF faculty. One-third of all faculty disclosures involved paid consulting arrangements providing up to $120,000 per year. Of the individuals who received industry money for consulting, more than half (61%) received less than $10,000 annually.

Benefits of Government-Industry Relationships

The benefits of GIRs are probably similar to those associated with AIRs. Relationships that foster more interaction among scientists with shared goals are likely to enhance creativity and productivity, and there can be little doubt that financial incentives are effective motivators of individual and organizational behaviors. To the extent that these relationships can speed the development of new discoveries and technological advances, society may benefit. As noted earlier, however, to believe that these goals can be achieved without the potential for abuse by some in the system is probably naive.

Although government agencies receive some compensation for the use of their intellectual property, the financial benefits of such relationships most likely flow primarily to the companies and the government scientists involved in these relationships. Indeed, the primary financial benefit of GIRs is likely to be personal compensation. The series of newspaper articles about the NIH, described above, identified hundreds of consulting relationships between senior NIH officials and industry, totaling millions of dollars (Willman 2004). The public also may benefit from some GIRs, however, to the extent that these relationships enhance the ability of government to retain the finest scientists for its stewardship of the public investment in science.

Risks Associated with Industry Relationships

In recent years, much has been written about the potential risks associated with AIRs and GIRs (Bowie 1994; Angell 2000; Bodenheimer 2000; Krimsky 2003). Derek Bok (1994, 118), the former president of Harvard University, articulated the risks of industry relationships when he wrote that "relationships may divert the faculty. Graduate students may be drawn into projects in ways that sacrifice their education for commercial gain. Research performed with an eye toward profit may lure investigators into conflicts of interest or cause them to practice forms of secrecy that hamper scientific progress. Ultimately, corporate ties may undermine the university's reputation for objectivity."

Secrecy in Science

Openness is, or perhaps was, a fundamental norm underlying the social structure of academic science. However, there is strong evidence supporting the belief that relationships with industry are compromising this norm (Blumenthal et al. 1997; Campbell et al. 2002). Data from a national survey of genetics researchers and other life scientists showed that those with research funding from industry were significantly more likely to delay publication of their research results by more than six months to allow for the commercialization of their research (Campbell et al. 2002). Such delays may be problematic in rapidly advancing fields characterized by intense competition among labs for a common scientific achievement (such as genetic sequencing), as well as for individual scientists who may continue to work on problems that have already been solved, resulting in a waste of scientific resources—including time and tax dollars.

Bias in the Reporting of Research Results

A significant body of research now suggests that relationships between academic scientists and industry affect the propensity and content of scientific reports emerging from the industry-supported research. A meta-analysis of twenty-three studies on the impact of AIRs on the outcomes of science found "a statistically significant relationship between industry sponsorship and pro industry conclusions" (Bekelman, Li, and Gross 2003, 454). Scientific areas in which industry-funded studies led to pro-industry conclusions included randomized clinical trials in multiple myeloma, economic analyses of oncology drugs, nicotine and cognitive performance, nonsteroidal anti-inflammatory drugs, and calcium channel blockers. This association does not show that industry-funded research is intentionally biased toward pro-industry findings. It may be that industry selectively funds research likely to yield favorable conclusions or that industry-funded studies address different questions than non-industry-funded studies. Nevertheless, the association between AIRs and pro-industry results exceeds what would be expected from chance alone.

Adverse Effects on Education and Training

Another risk mentioned by Bok (2003) was that research relationships with industry might adversely affect scientists-in-training. Support for this concern can be found in a 1985 survey of 693 advanced trainees in the life sciences at six universities, which found that 34 percent of respondents whose faculty advisor(s) were supported by industry felt constrained in discussing their research results with other scientists (Gluck, Blumenthal, and Stoto 1987). This study also found that graduate students and postdoctoral fellows whose projects were supported by industry reported significantly fewer publications, on average (2.62), than those with no industry support (3.67). To date, there has been no subsequent national study of the effects of AIRs, positive or negative, on the educational activities of universities.

Shifting University Research Agendas

With all the benefits of AIRs and GIRs listed above (especially those involving personal compensation), several commentaries have expressed the worry that financial incentives will shift university science away from basic research and toward more applied, commercial projects (e.g., Bok 2003). There is little evidence to confirm such a hypothesis. Annual surveys by the National Science Foundation (NSF) do not suggest that the fundamental activities in university research and development have changed much, with the ratio of basic to applied research and development remaining stable at about 3:1 (National Science Foundation, Division of Science Resources Statistics 2004). In one study of more than thirty-four hundred faculty at six research universities in the 1980s and 1990s, the proportion of research dedicated to basic science did not alter over the two decades, even though licensing activity at those universities increased by an order of magnitude (Thursby and Thursby 2004).

Financial Conflicts of Interest

In this chapter, we define a financial conflict of interest (FCOI) as a state in which primary professional interests conflict with one or more secondary interests of a financial nature (Thompson 1993). Applying this definition to scientists and administrators requires an examination of what their primary and secondary interests are. For academic scientists, the primary interests are the search for understanding of biological processes and communication of that understanding to the research community and, in many instances, the education of the next generation of scientists. An additional primary interest for physicians in academic health centers—defined as medical schools and their owned or affiliated teaching hospitals and faculty—is providing patient care. For administrators of government and academic scientific organizations, the primary interest is leadership of the organization to facilitate the work of scientists. All other interests are secondary, including fostering institutional or personal financial gain, enhancing one's professional status, gaining power, or garnering recognition.

These secondary interests, and any conflicts between these secondary interests and an individual's or institution's primary interests, are not, in themselves, improper. As stated by the editors of *JAMA*, "Conflicts of interest are considered ubiquitous and inevitable in academic life, indeed, in all professional life" (DeAngelis, Fontanerosa, and Flanagin 2001, 89). In fact, secondary interests are often approved, and in some cases encouraged, by institutions (such as consulting services or faculty ownership of equity in a company stemming from an individual's research). They often exist as a byproduct of a researcher's primary interest and, as shown above, can provide benefits such as resources (e.g., research funding or gifts from industry) to enhance the pursuance of the researcher's primary mission.

Numerous examples of FCOIs exist in the modern scientific enterprise. These include scientists' ownership of equity in firms that could directly benefit financially from the results of their research; scientific administrators' relationships with companies that could directly benefit financially from research by individuals whom the administrators supervise; payment of scientists to promote company products and services at professional meetings; and bonus payments to clinical scientists for meeting enrollment goals in clinical trials. This is not an exhaustive list but is illustrative of the types of FCOI that can exist.

Both relationships between industry and academic institutions or academic researchers and relationships between industry and government or government researchers can generate FCOIs. For many individuals and organizations, the mere perception of an FCOI is seen as problematic. Individuals and organizations holding such views may fail to understand that some FCOIs are inevitable and simply result from the structure of science, rather than representing a breaking of the rules or some form of misconduct.

Misconduct

The mere presence of an FCOI often generates distrust and suspicion of the academic and government research communities. Yet these FCOIs amount to misconduct (including bias) only when the pursuit of an individual's primary interests is superseded by a financial secondary interest. Examples of FCOIs that amount to misconduct include, but are not limited to, scientists engaging in research misconduct (e.g., falsification of data; giving inappropriately poor reviews to papers under consideration at a national journal) because doing so will financially benefit themselves or a company with which they have an interest; physicians enrolling ineligible patients in a clinical trial to boost the amount of money received for patient recruitment; individuals thwarting a study sponsored by a competitor of a company with which they have an interest; scientists consciously presenting information in a biased manner to influence the audience toward a product or service offered by a company with which they have an interest; and university administrators giving preferential contracts to a firm with which they have an interest.

Instances of such misconduct are believed to be relatively rare in the current scientific environment. There are several possible explanations for this. For example, institutional and government policies on FCOIs, such as those provided by the Association of American Medical Colleges (AAMC) and other groups, may limit the extent of misconduct. Also, the culture of science and the prevailing normative practices may successfully discourage such behavior. It is also possible, however, that mechanisms to detect the frequency and severity of misconduct in academic science are ineffective. Unfortunately, comprehensive, empirical data do not yet exist to address this question.

Implications for Government-Industry Relationships

The concrete risks of GIRs are likely to be similar to those of AIRs, but elected officials and the public may perceive GIRs as more problematic because the participants are government employees. Because the NIH and other federal research funding agencies have the primary responsibility for managing the public investment in science, openness and disclosure of GIRs are essential. One can make a case that these reporting requirements must be at least as stringent as those in place for academic institutions, as they currently are.

Current Policies and Practices on the Disclosure and Management of Industry Relationships

Efforts to disclose and manage AIRs take several forms, ranging from reliance on unwritten academic norms to general university policies and explicit federal regulations. Academic norms tend to support principles such as academic freedom, freedom of publication, and university control of research direction and outcomes (Merton 1968). A compelling case can be made, however, that norms alone have not proved effective in managing the risks of AIRs and GIRs, as both academic and government scientists have actively resisted the strengthening of prohibitions against establishing financial relationships with industry, even when those relationships pose clear and problematic conflicts of interest.

Public Health Service and FDA Regulations

The public sector has long complemented institutional culture and norms with explicit regulation of AIRs. Government agencies such as the Public Health Service (PHS) agencies and the NSF have had established regulations on individual FCOIs since 1995, including conflicts on the part of university officials in research sponsored by these agencies. The regulations require institutions to have in place policies and procedures that necessitate disclosure of some, but not all, relationships with industry and to take appropriate action to manage or eliminate the conflict before the expenditure of federal research funds.

Specifically, PHS policy requires that all industry relationships that may affect PHS-funded research and that result in the receipt of more than $10,000 annually or 5 percent of the total equity in a company must be disclosed to university officials. The nature of such relationships need not be reported to the federal agencies—the agencies just need to be informed that a conflict of interest was identified and managed or eliminated. Operationally, this puts the burden of management solely on the institution rather than the government, and accordingly, institutions bear any costs and risks associated with this oversight.

In 1998, the FDA adopted its own set of rules for disclosing and managing FCOIs on the part of external parties. These rules require that investigators who receive compensation in excess of $25,000 from a corporate sponsor of a trial in which they are engaged must disclose the relationship to the FDA, but not until the study has been completed and a marketing approval application for a drug, device, or biologic is filed. If the FDA determines that the relationship may have undermined the objectivity of the data, the agency may decline to accept those data in support of the marketing approval application. The threat that the FDA will reject data is probably sufficient to dissuade most investigators and companies from using investigators with FCOIs, but disclosure or elimination of conflicting relationships before launching a trial might be more effective in preserving research quality than the threat of data rejection alone.

Rules for NIH Employees

On February 1, 2005, the U.S. Department of Health and Human Services announced rules for all senior government scientists, including the six thousand senior scientists at the NIH, regarding financial interests that result from consulting relationships, equity relationships, and gift relationships. As a result, government scientists are prohibited from working for any biotechnology, pharmaceutical, medical device, or similar company, regardless of whether the firm is directly related to their individual duties. Other types of external relationship are also forbidden, including working with hospitals, health providers, health insurers, health-research-related trade organizations, and even educational or research institutions that were recently NIH funding applicants, grantees, or contractors. Senior employees can no longer hold stock in any medical technology firm and are required to divest within 150 days (with other employees subject to a $15,000 cap on holdings). Finally, government scientists cannot accept awards or gifts greater than $200 in value, with the possible exception of the Nobel or Lasker prizes. Recognizing that this new regulation falls at the more conservative end of the policy spectrum, NIH Director Elias A. Zerhouni commented: "Though I believe that some outside activities are in the best interest of the public when designed to accelerate the development of new discoveries, we must first have better oversight systems to ensure transparency and sound ethical practices and procedures" (National Institutes of Health, Office of the Director 2005a, 1).

Guidelines and Recommendations

In addition to the dramatic move by the NIH, several professional organizations—notably, the AAMC and the Association of American Universities—have taken leadership positions in the debate about AIRs in clinical research by developing explicit policy positions. The AAMC Task Force on Financial Conflicts of Interest in Clinical Research (2001) made the following recommendations (among others):

- Institutions should have a standing institutional conflict-of-interest committee or process.
- Institutions should adopt mechanisms to ensure that disclosures are readily accessible in the institution.
- Institutions should have clearly defined, written policies on financial interests in clinical research.
- Most important, in all research involving human subjects, institutions should begin with a presumption that for both investigators and institutions, no financial relationships that could compromise the interests or well-being of the participants will be tolerated and that this presumption may be rebutted, but only under compelling circumstances.

Currently, the impact of the AAMC and other policies and practices on the disclosure and management of AIRs is unclear. While almost all major research universities have a process for disclosure, there is great variation among institutional policies and practices in this area. A content analysis of the conflict-of-interest policies at the hundred universities that received the most NIH funding in 1998 found that the disclosure policies varied widely. For example, 55 percent of the policies required disclosures from all faculty members, while

45 percent required only principal investigators to disclose. Fewer than 20 percent of institutional policies specified limits on faculty financial relationships with industry, and 12 percent provided specific limits on the amount of time publications could be delayed (Cho et al. 2000). In addition, the fact that universities have policies and practices on the disclosure and management of relationships does not mean that these policies are enforced or that they are effective in preventing misconduct. A survey of the conflict-of-interest policies at U.S. institutions receiving more than $5 million in funding from the NIH or NSF found that the management of conflicts and penalties for nondisclosure were almost universally discretionary (Bekelman, Li, and Gross 2003).

Suggestions for Policy and Management

Based on the data presented in this chapter, we believe that the modern scientific enterprise comprises a set of complex, deeply integrated financial relationships among government, industry, and university-based scientists and their organizations. These relationships have benefits for individual scientists, their institutions, and the overall progress of science. However, these relationships also carry risks that cannot and should not be ignored, including, but not limited to, risks of misconduct, increased secrecy, and bias in the reporting of research results. The risks, like the benefits, exist for all faculty members who conduct academic activities, including research, teaching, and (for some) patient care, not just those who conduct clinical research. The existence of both risks and benefits suggests that an optimal strategy for both government and academia would be to manage GIRs and AIRs in such a way as to minimize the risks while preserving these beneficial relationships. A general approach to managing GIRs and AIRs should involve disclosure of all such relationships relevant to private and public authorities, identification and elimination of relationships that pose, a priori, unacceptable risks, and careful monitoring of relationships where the benefits are seen to outweigh the risks.

Standardizing Disclosure Policies for Academic-Industry Relationships

At present, as we have seen, there is wide variation in the disclosure policies and practices at universities, and perhaps even more variation in their application. Almost all universities have a mechanism for the disclosure of

AIRs. However, institutions differ greatly in who must disclose. Critics view the paucity (or lack) of measures in place to discover relationships that are not voluntarily disclosed, as well as the inconsistency in holding individuals accountable for nondisclosure, as a serious weakness of the current approach—which, some have argued, can only euphemistically be described as an oversight system.

To avoid the potential for institutions to benefit from having low standards for disclosure of AIRs, we suggest that the academic community develop and adopt harmonized, uniform policies covering the disclosure of these relationships. The policies should include a requirement for all faculty who conduct research or teach, as well as all institutional administrators at the level of department chair and above, to disclose their financial relationships with industry (including those of immediate family members) to a committee designated to receive and review such disclosures. To remedy the variations in which relationships must be disclosed, we suggest that universities require annual disclosure of all licensing, consulting, honoraria, and gift relationships that have an annual value of $10,000 or more and are related to an individual's area of professional expertise. Universities should also require annual disclosure of all equity relationships (excluding equity held as part of a mutual fund, part of a blind trust, etc.) held by individual faculty and senior administrators (or immediate family members) that are valued at $10,000 or more or that represent more than 5 percent of stock in companies related to an individual's area of professional expertise.

Independent Review of Financial Disclosures

It is the responsibility of academic institutions to carefully review the disclosures of faculty and administrators. The PHS requires institutions to designate a single individual to review disclosures related to PHS-funded research. However, because most major universities have a large number of faculty members who would be required to disclose under the suggestions outlined above, and because of the complex nature of certain relationships, disclosures should be reviewed by a formal committee that is adequately staffed. Further, to provide a measure of transparency similar to the review of clinical research protocols by IRBs, all disclosures should be reviewed and approved by an independent review committee made up of members from the institution and the local communities, similar to the structure of IRBs.

A content review of the disclosure policies at all medical schools in the

United States and the 170 institutions that received more than $5 million in funding from the NSF found that in almost every instance, penalties for non-disclosure were totally discretionary and uniformly nonspecific (McCrary et al. 2000). Therefore, we suggest that all institutions establish specific, meaningful, mandatory penalties for failing to disclose relationships with industry as specified by institutional policies.

Institutional Oversight and Management of Academic-Industry Relationships

Given the wide variation among universities in the frequency of certain types of AIR, in the institutions' organizational structure, and in academic decision-making processes, it is important to vest significant institutional discretion in the review and oversight of AIRs at the local level. Institutions should have some flexibility to decide which relationships require oversight and how to design, implement, and evaluate institutional oversight plans and activities.

Currently, the federal government has done little to assist institutions in this regard. According to a review article (Henderson and Smith 2002), government controls on FCOIs convey an overlapping, incomplete, and occasionally conflicting message to investigators and institutions involved in partnerships with industry, making compliance difficult and creating the potential for considerable variation in actual policy at the local level. Universities should receive clear, unambiguous guidance from the federal government concerning their responsibilities for ensuring the integrity of research and the protection of human subjects in the context of AIRs.

There is, as yet, no comprehensive source of data on the oversight activities of universities, beyond the case study at the University of California, San Francisco (Boyd and Bero 2000). Without data, it is difficult for institutions to learn from themselves or from one another in this area. Thus, aggregate, de-identified data on annual disclosures by faculty members and senior administrators (including a summary of the decisions of institutional oversight committees regarding these relationships) should regularly be made public.

In all publicly funded research, the activities and relationships of investigators or institutions that (1) are considered to represent FCOIs within applicable federal policies and guidance and (2) are allowed, after appropriate review and consideration, for compelling reasons, should be openly disclosed to the funding agency and the public. Disclosure should consist of (1) a detailed explanation of the rationale for determining that a compelling interest exists for allowing the work to proceed in spite of the conflict and (2) a description of the measures that will be taken to protect the interests, safety, and well-being of those whose interests are at stake.

The most recent data available suggest that 12 percent of universities provide specific limits on the amount of time publications may be delayed in the context of faculty members' relationships with industry (Cho et al. 2000). To ensure that scientific findings are published in a timely manner and to allow sufficient time to protect intellectual property in science, we suggest that institutions adopt a uniform policy that prohibits suppression of data. The FDA and corporate sponsors of clinical trials should adopt and adhere to a policy that the results of clinical trials, regardless of outcome, must be made available to the public in an appropriate format.

Given the amount of research in most universities and its highly technical nature, we believe the responsibility for protecting the integrity of scientific publications and presentations rests primarily with the investigators leading the research efforts. All authors should fully disclose all AIRs, in addition to the sources of research funding, related to a journal publication, according to the guidelines outlined above. In addition, at conferences or professional meetings, all presenters should fully disclose all AIRs, in addition to the sources of research funding, related to a presentation, according to the guidelines outlined above. Finally, ghostwriting of manuscripts by industrial sponsors of research or their agents in the name of an academic scientist or scientists must be understood as contrary to principles of responsible conduct and as a flagrant violation of professional standards of authorship for scientific publication; such practices are unacceptable and should be specifically prohibited.

Review of Government-Industry Relationships

As we have demonstrated, there is a substantial corpus of empirical data, collected primarily through large national surveys and case studies, showing that AIRs in the life sciences are a fundamental part of the modern life sciences enterprise. These data—which are now relatively old—have supported the development and implementation of policies and practices of individual universities, scientific journals, and professional associations to address the risks associated with industry relationships. However, while we know that government scientists and administrators comprise an important part of the life sciences enterprise and that they also have relationships with industry

(Willman 2004), there are no comprehensive, publicly available data to illuminate the risks and benefits of GIRs.

Such studies are both desirable and possible. Two sources of data are apparent. The first could be through case studies and anonymous surveys of government scientists and administrators in federal agencies such as the NIH, NSF, FDA, and others. A second potential source is the annual disclosure forms filed by federal employees. These forms, deidentified if necessary, should be made available for analysis. Using these data sources, appropriate organizations should systematically review the nature and extent of GIRs and release the deidentified results to the public.

The regulations promulgated by the NIH represent a sharp departure from the disclosure-based guidelines we recommend here, but they are largely consistent with the AAMC guidelines. It is important to gauge the impact of such rules, from the direct effect of reducing the number of GIRs to the potential unintended consequences of scientific migration out of the NIH, and the independence and objectivity of such an assessment must be unquestionable. Accordingly, an evaluation of the NIH's moratorium should be conducted by an organization independent of the federal government.

Review of Selected National Policies

As we have seen, AIRs carry significant benefits as well as risks. Two of the major stimuli for AIRs and GIRs were the Bayh-Dole Act and the Stevenson-Wydler Act, both passed in 1980. These policies have now been in place for more than a quarter of a century, with no comprehensive review to see whether changes could increase the productivity of AIRs and GIRs for the nation's economy and public health. The impact of the federal legislation that underlies the nation's efforts to commercialize life sciences research, including the Bayh-Dole and Stevenson-Wydler acts, should be reviewed by appropriate organizations to determine whether modifications might improve the effectiveness of technology transfer from the academic and government sectors to industry.

Conclusion

The prevalence and complexity of relationships among academia, government, and industry are likely to continue to grow and evolve in the years ahead. While the prospect for good to come from these relationships is real, so is the possibility of harm. We must continually look for new approaches to ensure the integrity and objectivity of science and protect the well-being of research participants.

At present, relationships between academic and government scientists and industry are a fundamental part of the modern life sciences enterprise and should not be eliminated. However, the benefits of these relationships should not be overstated, nor the risks ignored. The research findings thus far, as presented here, provide for only a limited ability to intelligently sort the risks associated with academic-industry and government-industry relationships. Under the tenet that "you manage what you measure," we have argued for more information and disclosure regarding the prevalence and magnitude of industry affiliations. Although disclosure of relationships with industry is common, if not universal, some standardization of the disclosure and management processes is desirable. Failure to do so could compromise the integrity and fundamental norms underlying the social structure of the modern life sciences enterprise.

ACKNOWLEDGMENTS

The views expressed are those of the authors alone and do not necessarily represent the views of Harvard Medical School, Partners HealthCare, the Institute for Health Policy, or the Ewing Marion Kauffman Foundation.

This work was supported by a research grant from the Ewing Marion Kauffman Foundation, Kansas City, Missouri. The foundation works with partners to advance entrepreneurship in the United States and improve the educational achievement of youth. The foundation's interest in helping to propagate new ideas and advance entrepreneurship has resulted in a focused view of the specific processes of innovation creation and commercialization. The late entrepreneur Ewing Marion Kauffman established the foundation in the mid-1960s. Information about the Kauffman Foundation is available at www.kauffman.org.

The work reported here was presented at the American Enterprise Institute–Brookings Joint Center for Regulatory Studies, Washington, DC, June 10, 2004 (www.aei-brookings.org). An abbreviated version of this chapter was published as E. G. Campbell, G. Koski, D. E. Zinner, and D. Blumenthal, "Managing the triple helix in the life sciences," *Issues in Science and Technology*, Winter (2005): 48–54.

AUTHOR DISCLOSURES

In 2003–4, E. G. Campbell received more than $10,000 in consulting income for research services provided to the Panel of Life Science Advisors of the Kauffman Foundation, under subcontract to the George Washington University. G. Koski is an unpaid member of the board of trustees of the American Academy of Pharmaceutical Physicians and the Association of Clinical Research Professionals.

References

AAMC Task Force on Financial Conflicts of Interest in Clinical Research. 2001. *Protecting Subjects, Preserving Trust, Promoting Progress: Policy and Guidelines for the Oversight of Individual Financial Interests in Human Subjects Research.* Washington, DC: Association of American Medical Colleges.

Angell, M. 2000. Is academic medicine for sale? *New England Journal of Medicine* 342 (20): 1516–18.

Bekelman, J. E., Y. Li, and C. P. Gross. 2003. Scope and impact of financial conflicts of interest in biomedical research. *JAMA* 289 (4): 454–65.

Blumenthal, D., E. G. Campbell, M. S. Anderson, N. Causino, and K. S. Louis. 1997. Withholding of research results in academic life science: Evidence from a national survey of faculty. *JAMA* 277 (15): 1224–28.

Blumenthal, D., E. G. Campbell, N. Causino, and K. S. Louis. 1996. Participation of life-science faculty in research relationships with industry. *New England Journal of Medicine* 335 (23): 1734–39.

Blumenthal, D., N. Causino, E. G. Campbell, and K. S. Louis. 1996. Relationships between academic institutions and industry in the life sciences: An industry survey. *New England Journal of Medicine* 334 (6): 368–73.

Bodenheimer, T. 2000. Uneasy alliance: Clinical investigators and the pharmaceutical industry. *New England Journal of Medicine* 342 (20): 1539–44.

Bok, D. 1994. The commercialized university. In *University-Business Partnerships: An Assessment,* ed. N. Bowie. Lanham, MD: Rowman & Littlefield.

———. 2003. *Universities in the Marketplace: The Commercialization of Higher Education.* Princeton, NJ: Princeton University Press.

Bowie, N. 1994. *University-Business Partnerships: An Assessment.* Lanham, MD: Rowman & Littlefield.

Boyd, E., and L. Bero. 2000. Assessing faculty financial relationships with industry: A case study. *JAMA* 284 (17): 2209–14.

Campbell, E. G., D. Blumenthal, and K. S. Louis. 1998. Looking a gift horse in the mouth: Corporate gifts that support life sciences research. *JAMA* 279 (13): 995–99.

Campbell, E. G., B. R. Clarridge, M. Gokhale, L. Birenbaum, S. Hilgartner, N. A. Holtzman, and D. Blumenthal. 2002. Data-withholding in academic genetics: Evidence from a national survey. *JAMA* 287 (4): 473–81.

Campbell, E. G., T. J. Weissman, S. Feibelmann, B. Moy, and D. Blumenthal. 2004. Institutional academic industry relationships: Results of case studies. *Accountability in Research* 11 (2): 103–18.

Cho, M. K., R. Shohara, A. Schissel, and D. Rennie. 2000. Policies on faculty conflicts of interest at US universities. *JAMA* 284 (17): 2203–8.

Cohen, J. 2005. AAMC strongly endorses NIH ban on outside activities. Association of American Medical Colleges. Press release, Feb. 2. www.aamc.org/newsroom/pressrel.

Cohen, W. M., R. R. Nelson, and J. P. Walsh. 2002. Link and impacts: The influence of public research on industrial R&D. *Management Science* 48 (1): 1–23.

DeAngelis, C. D., P. B. Fontanerosa, and A. Flanagin. 2001. Reporting financial conflicts of interests and relationships between investigators and research sponsors. *JAMA* 288 (1): 89–91.

Fox, M. F. 1985. Publication, performance and reward in science and scholarship. In *Higher Education: Handbook of Theory and Research*, 1:255–382, ed. J. C. Smart. New York: Agathon Press.

Gluck, M., D. Blumenthal, and M. A. Stoto. 1987. University-relationships in the life sciences: Implications for students and post-doctoral fellows. *Research Policy* 16 (6): 327–66.

Grady, D. 2004. Medical research dealings explored by Senate panel. *New York Times*, Jan. 23.

Henderson, J. A., and J. J. Smith. 2002. Financial conflict of interest in medical research: Overview and analysis of federal and state controls. *Food and Drug Law Journal* 57 (3): 445–56.

Jones, L. M. 2000. The commercialization of academic science: Conflict of interest for the faculty consultant. Ph.D. diss, University of Minnesota.

Kauffman Foundation Scientific Advisory Committee. 2003. *Technology Transfer and Commercialization in the Life and Health Sciences.* Report prepared for Panel of Advisors on the Life Sciences, Ewing Marion Kauffman Foundation. Kansa City, MO: Ewing Marion Kauffman Foundation.

Krimsky, S. 2003. *Science in the Private Interest: Has the Lure of Profits Corrupted Biomedical Research?* Lanham, MD: Rowman & Littlefield.

Kush, R., K. Getz, A. Whalen, and M. Lamberti 2002. *Attitudes, Adoption, and Usage of Technologies for e-Clinical Trials/EDC and Data Interchange Standards.* Boston: Clinical Data Interchange Standards Consortium–CenterWatch.

Marshall, E. 2003. Zerhouni pledges review of NIH consulting in wake of allegations. *Science* 302 (5653): 2046.

McCrary, S. V., C. B. Anderson, J. Jakovljevic, T. Khan, L. B. McCullough, N. P. Wray, and B. Brody. 2000. A national survey of policies on disclosure of conflicts of interest in biomedical research. *New England Journal of Medicine* 343 (22): 1621–26.

Merton, R. F. 1968. *Social Theory and Social Structure.* New York: Free Press.

National Institutes of Health, Office of the Director. 2005a. NIH announces sweeping ethics reform. Press release, Feb. 1. www.nih.gov/news.

———. 2005b. NIH calls on scientists to speed public release of research publications: Online archive will make articles accessible to the public. Press release, Feb. 3. www.nih.gov/news.

National Science Foundation, Division of Science Resources Statistics. 2004. *Academic Research and Development Expenditures: Fiscal Year 2002.* NSF 04-330. Project officer, M. Marge Machen. Arlington, VA: National Science Foundation.

Thompson, D. F. 1993. Understanding financial conflicts of interest. *New England Journal of Medicine* 329 (8): 573–76.

Thursby, J. G., and M. C. Thursby. 2004. Intellectual property: University licensing and the Bayh-Dole act. *Science* 303 (5654): 40.

Willman, D. 2004. Probe sought into NIH officials' outside work. *Los Angeles Times*, Jan. 17.

PART II

LEARNING FROM OTHER FIELDS

CHAPTER 5

Conflict of Interest in Financial Services

A Contractual Risk-Management Analysis

JOHN R. BOATRIGHT, PH.D.

As a moral concept, conflict of interest has a generally accepted meaning that can be applied in a wide range of settings. A comprehensive book, *Conflict of Interest in the Professions* (Davis and Stark 2001), contains chapters on conflicts in areas as diverse as law, medicine, government, engineering, business, journalism, and academics. Despite this common definition, however, the situations that constitute a conflict of interest, the reasons that conflicts are morally objectionable, and the means for addressing such conflicts vary greatly. Still, much can be learned from comparing conflicts of interest in different fields. This chapter examines conflicts of interest in financial services to shed light on possible approaches to understanding and managing conflicts in biomedical research. The financial services considered here include those offered by such institutions as banks, mutual funds, brokerage firms, insurance companies, and financial advisors, to both individual and corporate clients.

I have offered elsewhere a comprehensive survey of conflicts of interest in financial services (Boatright 2001), where I observe that conflicts of interest arise primarily because financial service providers serve as agents or intermediaries in executing investors' financial transactions and as fiduciaries or custodians in safeguarding their assets. Conflicts of interest are built into the structure of our financial institutions, because these institutions typically provide multiple services to multiple clients. Although some conflicts can and perhaps should be reduced, others are difficult to eradicate without forgoing the benefits of large, comprehensive financial institutions. The main challenge in the financial services industry, therefore, is to manage conflicts of interest with such means as adequate disclosure and effective rules and policies.

In this chapter, I go beyond my previous work and provide an analysis of conflict of interest in financial services as a risk-management problem. In doing so, I am building on a distinction made by lawyer Kevin McMunigal (2001) between two kinds of conflict-of-interest rules in the legal profession—namely, rules for preventing harm and rules for reducing risk. Generally speaking, the approach in the professions, especially medicine and law, has been to protect patients and clients against any harm from conflicts, primarily by adopting rules against acquiring adverse interests. However, it is not always possible, or even desirable, to seek the elimination of all harm. We brave many risks to enjoy greater gains. Investment, in particular, can never be risk free; indeed, risk is inversely correlated with return. The aim in financial services, therefore, is to manage risk prudently, including the risk that comes from conflicted financial service providers.

A Contractual Framework

Conflicts of interest in financial services differ from those in the professions in several important respects. First, with a few possible exceptions—financial advisors may be one—financial service providers are not professionals in the accepted sense of the term. In particular, they do not have what John Ladd (1997, 515) describes as an "altruistic orientation," in which the "commitment to the service of others and of society is paramount." As a result, self-interest plays a large and legitimate role in financial services. For example, a broker may be an agent and a fiduciary with respect to managing a client's account, but a broker may also deal with that same client in a buyer-seller relation, as, for example, when recommending certain securities.

Insofar as financial service providers are not professionals, the norms for their activities cannot be derived from their professional role. The prohibitions against conflict of interest in medicine and law, for example, are founded on the *structure* of a profession—that is, on what it means to be a physician or an attorney. By contrast, the norms for the conduct of financial service providers are derived from the *contracts* that they enter into. In other words, for financial service providers, it is the terms of financial contracts rather than the features of a professional role that determine the standards of acceptable behavior with respect to conflict of interest. Put simply, an attorney in a conflict-of-interest situation is not being a good attorney, whereas a conflicted broker, for example, is violating a contractual agreement with a customer.

The distinction between the terms of a contract and the structure of a profession might be regarded as one of degree, especially if professionals are viewed as having an unwritten contract with society. There is still a difference worth noting, however, because such a contract is made with society by professionals as a group, whereas the contract between a financial service provider and a client is between individuals or organizations and is subject to negotiation by these parties. That said, some of the duties of a broker, for example, are specified by law and are thus like the duties of professionals, to the extent that they are inherent in serving a particular role. However, other duties of a broker depend on the particular contractual arrangements that exist between firms and their customers.

Financial services consist mostly of contracting, which includes not only one-time transactions—such as an order to a broker to execute a trade—but also long-term relationships (Goetz and Scott 1981). For example, a homeowner with a mortgage enters into a relationship with a bank to make principal and interest payments over many years, and all securities are a kind of contract that commits two or more parties to certain obligations, often over an extended period of time. It is by means of contracting that we form economic organizations and institutions (Williamson 1985). Indeed, the dominant school of financial economics models the modern corporation as a nexus of contracts between the various corporate constituencies (Coase 1937; Jensen and Meckling 1976; Easterbrook and Fischel 1991).

In financial services contracting, it is assumed that all parties are self-interested and that each is deploying his or her assets to achieve the greatest risk-adjusted return. Such contracting in financial services creates risks of at least two kinds. One kind is the risk inherent in financial markets, as when an investor buys a stock that can decrease in value. This is *market risk.* A second kind of risk involves the contract between an investor and a financial service provider whereby the provider, who is the investor's agent, may not fulfill his or her obligations. This is commonly known as *agency risk.* Agency risk may result either from self-interested or opportunistic behavior by an agent or from the inability of an agent to serve all customers or clients (the principals) equally well. For example, when a broker must allot a security in short supply, a less-favored customer runs the risk of losing out.

Market risk is inherent in economic activity. Whether an investment succeeds depends on many factors that cannot be anticipated or controlled. Agency risk, by contrast, is due, in part, to the inability of the parties in an agency relationship to write fully specified contracts that detail the expected conduct of each party and the recourse each has for noncompliance. This is a condition known as *imperfect contracting*. Because of imperfect contracting, a financial service provider has a certain amount of discretion that creates risk for an investor. Some people in business may choose not to write fully specified, perfect contracts, even when such contracts are possible, because of cost or other factors (Macaulay 1963), but in many cases it is impossible to plan completely, which is a requirement of perfect contracts. The main obstacles to perfect contracting are *complexity, contingency,* and *uncertainty.* Thus, the standard reasons given for the inability of shareholders to write perfect contracts with managers are that the situations likely to be faced by managers are exceedingly complex (complexity), that not all situations can be foreseen (contingency), and that, even if they could be foreseen, shareholders may not know what should be done (uncertainty).

One solution to this inability to write perfect contracts is to impose fiduciary duties. A fiduciary duty, which is the duty of a person in a position of trust to act in the interests of another, solves the problems of complexity, contingency, and uncertainty by requiring a fiduciary to act as if he or she were in the position of the beneficiary. However, fiduciary duties create the conditions for conflicts of interest precisely because a fiduciary's own interest might interfere with his or her ability to act in the interests of this other party. Indeed, conflicts of interest arise only in situations such as agency and fiduciary relationships, where one person has an obligation to act in another's interest.

When contracts are imperfect, for whatever reason, the parties seek to protect themselves with various safeguards. The imposition of fiduciary duties on managers is a form of protection that partially solves the contracting problem that shareholders have with a firm. Many other kinds of safeguard or protection are possible. In an article on the theory of the firm (Boatright 2002), I offer a classification of the means by which various constituencies can seek to protect themselves in their relationship with a firm. One division is between means that rely on precise rules and market mechanisms to protect a group's interests and means that attempt to protect group interests by using legal and moral norms, such as fiduciary duties. I label these *contract* and *trust* approaches, respectively. These two kinds of means can be further categorized as those that apply on (1) the level of specific decisions, (2) the transaction level, at which contracts or other arrangements are formed, and (3) the level of the system.

For example, bondholders, who provide capital to a firm in return for a promise to repay the principal with interest, are at risk of reduced creditworthiness and default. Generally, bondholders seek to protect themselves with precise rules rather than relying, as shareholders do, on fiduciary duties; thus, the protections for bondholders use a contract rather than a trust approach. The contract between bondholders and the firm is contained mostly on the system level in the body of securities law and the Bankruptcy Code (which specifies bondholder rights in the event of insolvency). These systemic protections apply to every bondholder because they are a part of the legal framework. Consequently, bondholders do not have to negotiate these protections for each bond issue; these protections have already been put in place by legislators, precisely to avoid the need for bondholders to negotiate them each time. Protections on the transaction level include the terms or covenants of particular bond issues, which may be negotiated or, as is more often the case, are determined by the market. That is, the issuers of bonds are led by market forces to offer the terms that investors are thought to demand. Finally, bondholders may seek the power to influence specific corporate decisions—for example, by insisting on bond covenants that grant a right of veto over certain management decisions.

These two sets of distinctions can be expressed in a matrix (figure 5.1). The shading in the matrix indicates that corporate constituencies seek to protect themselves either by a contract approach on the system level (lower left corner) or by a trust approach on the decision level (upper right corner). The darker shading indicates greater reliance on means in these areas.

The arrows in figure 5.1 represent two further dimensions. First, sociologists make a distinction between informal systems of social control that are based on situational personal relationships and more formal systems of social control that regulate with universal, impersonal rules, often codified into law and enforced by state power. A second distinction, more often made by economists, is between systems of regulation that rely on market mechanisms as opposed to those that rely on personal responsibility. For example, pollution can be regulated either by imposing a legal and perhaps a moral duty on managers to reduce pollution (a responsibility approach) or by creating market mechanisms, such as a market for pollution rights (a market approach). In general, safeguards in the lower left corner of the matrix constitute more formal systems of social control that use market mechanisms, while those in the

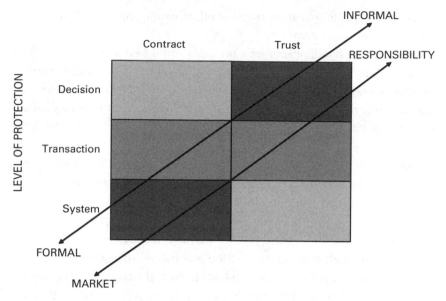

Figure 5.1. Means for protecting constituency interests.

upper right corner exemplify informal systems of social control that employ personal responsibility.

Figure 5.1 can be used to understand the safeguards or protections sought by the various constituencies that are assumed to contract with a nexus-of-contracts firm. Among the implications of this model are that the safeguards chosen are themselves the result of bargaining and that each has costs that must be weighed against the benefits. Thus, the constituencies that contract with a firm—among which are shareholders, bondholders, suppliers, customers, and employees—seek some combination of safeguards to protect themselves from the risk of participating in joint economic activity. The protections that they are able to achieve depend on the willingness of the firm to agree to the terms demanded by these constituencies, as in any market transaction. No group can be completely insulated from risk, and greater risk is voluntarily assumed only in return for greater benefits. For example, shareholders and bondholders are both investors in a firm, but shareholders, who assume greater risk, are rewarded with greater expected returns. Shareholders and bondholders can thus be viewed as groups that are alike in that each provides capital to a firm, but differ not only in the form of the expected return—that is, residual earnings profit as opposed to principal and interest payments—but also in the means for protecting their return and the risks they are willing to assume.

To summarize, financial services—indeed, most financial activities, including the creation of organizations and institutions—are commonly understood as systems of contracting. Financial contractors run the risk that the other party may not fulfill his or her obligations, especially when it is not possible to write perfect contracts. In such situations of imperfect contracting, the parties seek to protect themselves with various safeguards. Which safeguards are adopted depends on an evaluation of the costs and benefits of each safeguard and the willingness of the other party to agree to its adoption. The aim for any party is not to eliminate all risk—a goal that would be impossible as well as undesirable—but to manage the risk and achieve the desired risk-adjusted return. This contractual framework is useful for understanding the rules that protect shareholders, bondholders, suppliers, customers, and employees of a firm. The next step is to apply this framework specifically to the risk of conflict of interest in financial services.

A Market for Rules

When financial service providers serve as agents and fiduciaries, investors run the agency risk of loss due to conflicts of interest. Insofar as an investor can instruct a broker, for example, on what trades to make, the investor can write perfect contracts and thus exercise control. Such an investor may pay a price, however, by forgoing the opportunity to rely on a broker's knowledge and skill. An investor may often realize a greater return by giving the broker discretion to trade for that person's account. That return may be reduced, though, if the broker has a conflict of interest that leads him or her to put self-interest or the interest of other clients above that of the trusting investor. If this amount, known as *agency loss*, is less that the marginal gain that a broker can achieve by trading for the client, then the use of a conflicted agent is still worthwhile. The loss can be reduced, however, if the investor imposes rules on the broker with respect to conflict of interest. Alternatively, the broker may voluntarily adopt conflict-of-interest rules to assure brokerage customers—and perhaps to obtain a higher fee because of this assurance.

Conflict-of-interest rules can thus be understood as rules that reduce the agency risk to investors from financial service providers in their roles as agents and fiduciaries. This risk may result either from opportunistic, self-interested behavior or from having one's interests subordinated to those of others. For example, some brokers are offered higher compensation for recommending a firm's own mutual funds rather than the funds of independent mutual fund companies or competing investment banks (which might better serve a customer's needs). Similarly, securities analysts for some major banks have been accused of conflict of interest when the analysts' compensation is tied to their ability to facilitate the underwriting of securities offered by the firm. For example, in 2003, ten of Wall Street's largest firms paid $1.4 billion to settle charges that their top stock analysts had touted stocks of companies that brought their employers investment banking business, while denigrating these same companies in private communications (White and Day 2003). As part of the settlement, the firms also agreed to reinforce the walls that separate stock analysis from investment and to provide other sources of independent research. Because of conflicts of this type, some investors have bought stocks on the recommendation of analysts whose objectivity is compromised.

A conflict of interest also occurs when a financial service provider is pledged to serve the interests of more than one investor and cannot serve them all equally well. For example, investment banks often serve as advisors to a number of investment funds with similar investment objectives, such as investing in high-tech firms or emerging markets. These banks may also invest their own funds in the same kinds of venture. When limited investment opportunities present themselves, the bank must allot the securities among the various funds they advise and possibly their own funds. Under these conditions, no fund can be served as well as it would be if it were the bank's only client. A similar situation occurs when an investment bank has the opportunity to allot shares in an IPO (initial public offering). In the same $1.4 billion settlement previously cited, the ten Wall Street firms agreed to end the practice of offering shares of sought-after IPOs whose price is certain to rise quickly. The Securities and Exchange Commission (SEC) has held that offering shares of hot IPOs to favored executives of companies is an illegal gift, given to attract or retain those companies' business.

Unlike professionals, such as physicians and attorneys, financial service providers have little obligation, either moral or legal, to avoid conflicts of interest, except when these conflicts rise to the level of fraud. Legally and (arguably) ethically, a broker who is selling mutual funds may recommend an in-house fund that brings a higher commission without disclosing this fact to the investor, as long as the fund is suitable. Similarly, investment banks are not barred by law or ethics from advising multiple funds and making their own investments. Such conflicts are commonly understood and accepted by all funds that seek advice from investment banks. The objection to the allocation of IPOs to executives of client companies is not that it involves a conflict of interest but that the allocation appears to be a disguised kickback for bringing other business to the bank. Although accepting a kickback may compromise an executive's judgment and thus create a conflict of interest, it can also be a form of theft from the employing company, which is a wrong that is distinguishable from the harm of any compromised judgment.

All of these practices result in losses that investors may seek to prevent. For example, investors may not trust brokers who receive higher commissions for selling certain products, and they may be led, as a result, to seek out other, more trustworthy brokers. By exercising their rights in a market, investors may choose to deal only with brokers who do not have such a conflict of interest. Alternatively, brokers may seek to attract and retain customers by voluntarily avoiding conflict of interest. Investment banks may also seek to reassure client funds of their commitment to serve all of them equally well, and these funds may seek out advisors who have this commitment. In short, the adoption of rules concerning conflict of interest may be the subject of bargaining among investors and financial service providers. Such bargaining may take the form of explicit negotiations but is more likely to be a form of marketing in which financial service providers signal and attract investors with favorable terms. Whether the bargaining is explicit or implicit, the result is that conflict-of-interest rules are merely one more item for negotiation.

Conflict-of-interest rules in financial services may be understood, then, as safeguards that investors negotiate with financial service providers to reduce the risk of loss due to conflicts of interest. For example, some brokerage firms have responded to investors' concerns about higher compensation for in-house mutual funds by adopting a single rate for all funds. Major investment banks have agreed not to involve securities analysts in the bank's underwriting business and to separate analysts' compensation from the success of the business. Banks that advise funds often pledge to treat all funds that they advise equally or to clearly disclose the order of preference among funds. All of these measures are part of the contractual terms that financial service providers negotiate with investors in the marketplace.

This state of affairs may be described by saying that there is a market for conflict-of-interest rules. Such rules are like other economic goods, inasmuch as many different safeguards are possible; each has a cost as well as a benefit; and both investors and other parties involved must mutually agree on the adoption of any rules. Thus, a decision not to compensate brokers more for selling in-house funds bears a cost for brokerage firms, inasmuch as they make more money from such funds. However, investors may be willing to "buy" a rule that prohibits differential commissions, and firms may be willing to "sell" such a rule to investors to gain their business. In this case, both investors and firms realize that they are better off with the adoption of a rule under which there is no difference in commissions. The result is a market exchange or transaction.

Of course, conflict-of-interest rules are not the only safeguards available to investors, and other market transactions are possible. For example, an investor may avoid the need for conflict-of-interest rules by not giving a broker discretionary authority to trade for an account. The investor may also monitor a broker more carefully or may choose to invest only in independent mutual funds and thereby avoid the need for a broker's services entirely. However, as already noted, all of these options may be costly for an investor. Similarly, an investment fund may hire its own advisors rather than relying on the advisory services of an investment bank. Because these options exist, financial service providers have a great incentive to adopt rules that assure investors of uncompromised judgment.

Like any economic good, conflict-of-interest rules will be bought and sold only if what each party gives up is less than what it gains. Investors could, at a price, engage a broker who would provide exclusive service, in the way that a law client has the full attention of an attorney. Indeed, some wealthy investors have their own investment personnel, but for the average investor such exclusive service is impractical. As a result, brokers will have some conflicts of interest. The next question is, how much conflict is acceptable? Here the choice depends on the value of unconflicted service to an investor, which is a function of how much the investor stands to lose and the amount of risk the investor is willing to take.

If conflict-of-interest rules are like any other economic good, then investors will "buy" these rules and financial service firms will "sell" them, up to the point where the marginal benefit to each party exceeds their marginal cost. Moreover, conflict-of-interest rules are not a single kind of good but are more like items on a restaurant menu. Financial service providers can offer a certain range of safeguards to investors, and investors can choose the protections they prefer. As with other economic goods, investors may be satisfied with different packages of benefits and protections. Thus, investors may be indifferent in choosing between a low-commission broker with significant conflicts and a high-commission broker without such conflicts. In a competitive market, therefore, we would expect to find conflict-of-interest rules of varying kinds with different degrees of stringency that correspond to investors' preferences for particular rules and their willingness to assume risk.

In keeping with the idea of a market for conflict-of-interest rules, the actual rules that prevail will be determined by contracting among investors and financial service providers. They are, in other words, market choices that reflect the preferences of the contracting parties. This conclusion is sharply at variance with the usual conception of conflict of interest in the professions, according to which an avoidance of conflict of interest is an obligation or duty that a professional owes to a patient or client. This obligation or duty, moreover, is not based on contract, as it is in the provision of financial services, but has some moral ground that prohibits conflicts of interest for all professionals. Michael Davis offers an example of such a moral ground in his claim that being in a conflict-of-interest situation is morally wrong because it is a form of negligence, a betrayal of trust, and an impairment of competence (Davis 2001, 11–12). Assuming that Davis is right about why it is wrong to be in a conflict-of-interest situation, professionals are under an obligation to avoid conflicts. That is, the avoidance of conflict of interest is mandatory for all professionals.

The importance of the distinction between conflict-of-interest rules as contract-based and as morally grounded can be illustrated by fiduciary duties in corporate law, which are like conflict-of-interest rules in that they serve as safeguards in agency or trust relations against opportunistic behavior. Jonathan Macey (1999) observes that on the standard view, officers and directors have a mandatory fiduciary duty to shareholders that is supported by various moral arguments (many of these arguments are examined in Macey 1991). Macey argues, however, that "fiduciary duties are not what they appear to be," which is to say that they are not morally based obligations that are binding on all corporate officers and directors. He continues, "They can be (and frequently are) modified by contract" (Macey 1999, 1268). Thus, he characterizes fiduciary duties as protections that are bargained for among all of the constituencies in a nexus-of-contracts firm. They are usually assigned to shareholders only because shareholders seek them in their bargaining with the firm. Macey concludes that "contrary to popular wisdom, the notion that shareholders are the exclusive beneficiaries of fiduciary duties is the *default* rule rather than the *mandatory* rule" (1268). Insofar as they are embedded in law, then, conflict-of-interest rules are default, rather than mandatory, rules.

However, few conflict-of-interest rules in financial services are a matter of law. These rules are more commonly adopted voluntarily by financial service providers to meet investor demands. More important, most conflict-of-interest rules in financial services are not morally required but are the result of contracting between financial service providers and investors. They have moral (and sometimes legal) force, but only as rules agreed to in contracts.

Managing Conflict of Interest

Many means are available for managing conflict of interest. Aside from avoiding the acquisition of any interest that could interfere with serving the interests of another, the means include maintaining objectivity, making adequate disclosure, and referring decisions to persons with independent judgment. Competition can also be a strong counterforce to a personal interest. Bank trust departments, for example, compete on rates of return, so allocating brokerage business to firms that are bank customers—a practice known as reciprocation, or "recip"—will put that trust department at a competitive disadvantage if the broker cannot provide the best execution. In addition, a firm can make structural changes, such as separating lines of business that create a conflict—separating the trust department of a bank from the loan division, for example—and creating "Chinese walls" that control the flow of information (Boatright 2001).

Financial institutions rely primarily on rules and policies that work together to manage conflict of interest. Some rules and policies address conflicts directly through the means already noted, such as rules that forbid the acquisition of a competing interest or that require disclosure of a competing interest. Other rules and policies operate indirectly by preventing the acquisition of a competing interest or countering an existing interest. For example, investment banks have attempted to reduce conflicts of interest among securities analysts by policies that prohibit involving analysts in the solicitation of investment banking business and basing analysts' compensation on their contribution to this business. Rules and policies can be enforced more effectively when the relevant information is collected in a timely manner and analyzed by compliance officers and when there is high-level oversight, reaching even to the board of directors or the managing partners.

An example of the management of conflict of interest in the financial services industry is the regulation of personal investing by managers of mutual funds. This example is especially instructive because the problem of personal investing has been closely studied and detailed rules and procedures have been developed. The resulting system of regulation uses most of the available means for managing conflict of interest.

"Personal investing" refers to the situation in which the manager of a mutual fund invests in the same securities as the fund for his or her personal account. This situation creates a conflict of interest, first, because a fund manager has the opportunity to use *information* about impending fund transactions or about the securities to be bought or sold in his or her own trading. For example, a fund manager might make a personal trade in advance of a fund purchase, a practice known as front running. By engaging in front running, a fund manager can obtain securities with the expectation of a rise in price when they are purchased for the fund. A fund manager is also in possession of a great deal of securities analysis that belongs to the fund sponsor and should be used only for the benefit of the fund's shareholders.

A second source of conflict in personal investing is the opportunity to make *decisions* about fund transactions that benefit the fund manager's personal holdings. Thus, a manager might purchase a declining security for the fund to raise the price and thereby avoid a margin call in his or her own account. A fund manager might also receive some personal investment opportunity or other benefit in return for purchasing certain securities for the fund, or the manager might buy securities from or sell securities to the fund. Even if a fund manager does not take advantage of these opportunities, their existence undermines investors' confidence if the fund does not have rules and policies in place to prevent fund managers from taking personal advantage of their position.

The conflict of interest inherent in personal investing was recognized before the passage of the Investment Company Act in 1940. In 1966, the SEC studied the problem and requested that Congress grant the SEC the authority to regulate personal investing. In response, in 1970, Congress added section 17(j) to the Investment Company Act. In 1980, the SEC issued rule 17j-1, which is described below. Some violations of this rule in the 1990s prompted a review by the SEC and the Investment Company Institute (ICI), the industry association. The SEC report, *Personal Investment Activities of Investment Company Personnel,* was released in September 1994, preceded by the ICI report, *Report of the Advisory Group on Personal Investing,* in May 1994. These studies led the SEC to adopt amendments to rule 17j-1 in 1999.

Rule 17j-1, as promulgated in 1980, has four main components. First, the rule prohibits fraudulent, deceptive, or manipulative acts by "access persons" in their personal investments involving any securities held or to be acquired by the investment company. (An access person is anyone connected with a fund who may come across information on transactions by that fund or its clients in the regular course of his or her employment. This definition applies not only to managers of funds but also to employees of a fund's principal underwriter and investment advisor.) Second, the rule requires investment companies, along with their investment advisors and principal underwriters, to adopt codes of ethics containing provisions reasonably necessary to prevent access persons from engaging in prohibited fraudulent, deceptive, or manipulative acts. Third, access persons are required by the rule to report their personal securities transactions to their employer each quarter. Fourth, investment companies and their investment advisors and principal underwriters are required to maintain certain records, including quarterly transaction reports and codes of ethics, and to make these records available for inspection by the SEC. The 1999 amendments strengthened rule 17j-1 by requiring that (1) the boards of directors of funds assume greater responsibility to ensure compliance with the code; (2) access persons provide more information about their personal portfolio holdings; and (3) investment companies provide more information to the public about their rules and policies on personal investing.

Rule 17j-1 does not mandate any specific restrictions on personal investing by fund personnel or the adoption of specific procedures. Rather, decisions on these matters are left to each investment company in the belief that each company is in the best position to adopt rules and procedures that fit its situation. This delegation of responsibility, which is similar to federal rules for institutions receiving research funds from the government, also emphasizes that the organizations closest to the activity should have the primary responsibility for managing conflicts of interest and the flexibility to do it as they see fit. Investment companies have responded with detailed rules and procedures concerning prohibited transactions and required reports that apply to fund personnel, as well as detailed procedures to be followed by boards of directors in their oversight role.

The restrictions on personal investing by access persons generally consist of absolute prohibitions on certain transactions (such as IPOs, private placements, and short-term trading), blackout periods for trading in the same securities as the company (typically, seven days before and after a trade is made for the company), and requirements that certain transactions be precleared.

Preclearance is an important safeguard because fund managers may not be aware of trading activity in the rest of the company. Access persons are required by rule 17j-1 to submit a complete list of all securities held in their personal portfolios on joining the company and to update that list each year. In addition to filing quarterly reports of all transactions, access persons are required to certify annually that they have read the code and have complied with it. Access persons are further required to submit duplicate confirmation and account statements, to be sent directly from their brokers.

All of this submitted material is typically reviewed by a personal investment committee, which, in turn, issues annual reports to the board of directors that detail instances of improper trading activity and the sanctions imposed. The board of directors of a mutual fund is responsible for ensuring that sufficient rules and policies are in place to deter improper trading and that the system of regulation has been effective. As part of this responsibility, the board approves the codes of ethics and all material revisions, and it reviews annual reports of significant misconduct, including the sanctions imposed.

This system of regulation reflects a contractual framework, inasmuch as investors in mutual funds bear an agency risk when fund managers engage in personal investing, a risk that investors can seek to reduce by some means. Investors could seek out mutual funds managed by people who offer an exclusive loyalty in the manner of physicians and attorneys. Such unconflicted service is unlikely to be offered, however, because of the hardship that a prohibition on personal trading would place on fund managers. A prohibition on personal investing would also hinder mutual funds in attracting and retaining capable fund managers, which, in turn, would deny investors the benefit of their services. Thus, a certain level of conflict is in investors' interests, and investors and investment companies operating in a market would probably agree to rules that permit this level of conflict.

With respect to the choice of means represented in figure 5.1, most of the regulation of personal investing uses a contract approach on the transaction level, although rule 17j-1 is an example of regulation on the system level. Rule 17j-1 has some mandatory provisions, but for the most part it allows investment companies to experiment and to offer a variety of terms to investors. And investors who are concerned about the agency risk posed by personal investing can select mutual funds on the basis of the protections they offer. In this way, the determination of many specific features of the regulation of personal investing is left to the market—the market for rules.

Practical Implications

The example of the regulation of personal investing in the mutual fund industry provides some possible lessons about managing conflict of interest in other areas, including biomedical research. The following are merely suggestions that those more familiar with the conflicts in biomedical research can apply in appropriate ways.

1. *Gather data on the extent of conflicts and their seriousness.* No action should be taken until hard data show that conflicts of interest are sufficiently pervasive and serious to warrant action. In particular, it should not be assumed that conflicts are always wrong and must always be avoided. Rule 17j-1 was not adopted until extensive media reporting focused the attention of Congress and the public on the extent of abuses of trust in the mutual fund industry. Following these revelations, both the SEC and the ICI conducted thorough studies of personal investing before making recommendations for additional regulation. These studies found that the conflicts of interest in this activity were not serious enough to justify a complete ban but that more stringent rules were advisable. Among the benefits of such comprehensive studies are an industry consensus on the need for some action and a determination of what action is needed.

2. *Involve all of the relevant parties.* The regulation of personal investing has been addressed by Congress in enacting section 17(j); by the SEC in recommending that Congress act, in issuing a report on the problem (Securities and Exchange Commission 1994), and in issuing rule 17j-1; by ICI, the industry trade organization, in issuing its own report and in making recommendations to mutual fund companies (Investment Company Institute 1994); and by mutual fund companies themselves in adopting specific rules and policies. No one party is able to effectively regulate personal investing alone. In particular, the role of Congress is to set broad objectives, with implementation delegated to the SEC, a regulatory agency created by Congress specifically for this purpose. Although the SEC formulates and enforces rules, compliance is increased when these rules have broad acceptance by the industry and individual firms. Only by involving all of the relevant parties can rules be formulated in a process that allows for the representation of all interests, which is essential if there is to be a market for rules. The opportunity for each party to participate in the process of rule-making in a market inevitably involves compromise, but the outcome is more likely to be regulation that is acceptable to all parties and is thus more likely to be observed.

3. *Be flexible and allow for adaptation by those most closely involved.* A guiding principle of the SEC and ICI reports is that mutual fund companies can best provide oversight of personal investing by fund personnel by being given the flexibility to adopt rules and policies that are tailored to the companies' own circumstances. Rather than propose uniform standards for all mutual fund companies, these reports recommend that government and the industry association offer broad guidelines and leave implementation to the lowest level (the mutual fund company). For example, rule 17j-1 requires each company to adopt a code of ethics but does not specify any particular content. This kind of deference not only allows for flexibility but also permits companies to experiment to find the most effective means of regulation.

4. *Focus not merely on prohibiting certain conduct but also on ensuring compliance.* General principles and code provisions specify the conduct that is prohibited, but the rules and policies adopted should also aim to deter the prohibited conduct and detect noncompliance. Rule 17j-1 requires quarterly reports of all trading activity by fund managers, which are closely scrutinized by a firm's compliance staff. The reliability of this information is increased by a requirement that the compliance staff receive duplicate confirmation and account statements from an employee's broker. The compliance staff also receives requests for trades that require preclearance. The board of directors of a fund, which is charged with monitoring the code and ensuring that controls are in place, must receive annual reports of any material violations of the code and the sanctions imposed. Measures such as these increase managers' awareness of what conduct is prohibited and make detection of misconduct more likely. The important factors are reporting requirements that generate adequate data and high-level oversight that effectively uses these data.

5. *Have an appropriate mix of general principles and specific rules.* Much of the effectiveness of the regulation of personal investing derives from the detailed rules that most mutual fund companies have adopted. These rules include a precise specification of who is covered, a list of particular practices that are forbidden or that require preclearance, the timing of any blackout period during which certain trades are prohibited, and a clear explanation of exceptions to the rules. No set of rules can be complete, so general principles have a role in any regulatory system. However, the regulation of personal investing is more effective when the specifically prohibited behaviors are identified and addressed by rules.

6. *Communicate with all affected parties.* In the regulation of personal investing, it is most important for a mutual fund company to communicate to fund

managers the importance of avoiding improper personal investing and to inform them of the specific rules that govern their personal investment activities. This communication is achieved by requiring, in addition to quarterly reports of transactions, an annual report of all securities holdings and an annual signed statement of compliance with all rules and policies. Rule 17j-1 requires that a company's code of ethics be disclosed to the public and entered into EDGAR, the SEC's web-accessible database. Although additional disclosure is not legally mandated, some companies make details of their regulation of personal investing available to the public.

Conclusion

As characterized in this chapter, the management of conflict of interest in financial services is largely the search for means to reduce agency risk in investing. This risk cannot be eliminated entirely, and the reduction of risk beyond a certain point is undesirable. Nevertheless, investors seek some rules that reduce the risk posed by conflict of interest, and it is in the interest of financial service providers to offer these rules. Many means are available for reducing risk, and those in place are determined primarily by contracting in a market for rules. That is, investors seek to "buy" certain protections and financial service providers offer to "sell" them, so that the resulting system of regulation represents a kind of market equilibrium. This market for rules is exemplified by the regulation of personal investing in the mutual fund industry. I have attempted to draw some practical implications from this system of regulation that may be relevant to the management of conflict of interest in other areas. The applicability of these lessons to biomedical research is a question that I leave to the readers of this volume.

REFERENCES

Boatright, J. R. 2001. Financial services. In *Conflict of Interest in the Professions*, ed. M. Davis and A. Stark. New York: Oxford University Press.
———. 2002. Contractors as stakeholders: Reconciling stakeholder theory with the nexus-of-contracts firm. *Journal of Banking and Finance* 26 (9): 1837–52.
Coase, R. M. 1937. The nature of the firm. *Economica*, n.s., 4 (16): 386–405.
Davis, M. 2001. Introduction. In *Conflict of Interest in the Professions*, ed. M. Davis and A. Stark. New York: Oxford University Press.

Davis, M., and A. Stark, eds. 2001. *Conflict of Interest in the Professions*. New York: Oxford University Press.

Easterbrook, F. H., and D. R. Fischel. 1991. *The Economic Structure of Corporate Law*. Cambridge, MA: Harvard University Press.

Goetz, C. J., and R. E. Scott. 1981. Principles of relational contracts. *Virginia Law Review* 67 (6): 1089–1150.

Investment Company Institute. 1994. *Report of the Advisory Group on Personal Investing*. May 9. Washington, DC: Investment Company Institute.

Jensen, M. C., and W. H. Meckling. 1976. Theory of the firm: Managerial behavior, agency costs, and ownership structure. *Journal of Financial Economics* 3 (4): 305–60.

Ladd, J. 1997. Professional ethics. In *Blackwell Encyclopedia of Business Ethics*, ed. P. Werhane and R. Freeman. Malden, MA: Blackwell Publishers.

Macaulay, S. 1963. Non-contractual relations in business: A preliminary study. *American Sociological Review* 28 (1): 55–67.

Macey, J. R. 1991. An economic analysis of the various rationales for making shareholders the exclusive beneficiaries of corporate fiduciary duties. *Stetson Law Review* 21 (1): 23–44.

———. 1999. Fiduciary duties as residual claims: Obligations to nonshareholder constituencies from a theory of the firm perspective. *Cornell Law Review* 84 (5): 1266–81.

McMunigal, K. 2001. Conflict of interest as risk analysis. In *Conflict of Interest in the Professions*, ed. M. Davis and A. Stark. New York: Oxford University Press.

Securities and Exchange Commission. 1994. *Personal Investment Activities of Investment Company Personnel*. Sept. Washington, DC: Securities and Exchange Commission.

White, B., and K. Day. 2003. SEC approves Wall Street settlement: Conflicts of interest targeted. *Washington Post*, Apr. 29.

Williamson. 1985. *The Economic Institutions of Capitalism*. New York: Free Press.

CHAPTER 6

The Law and Ethics of Lawyers' Conflict of Interest

ROBERT LAWRY, J.D., L.L.M.

Conceptually, "conflict of interest" refers to the risk that actions taken or not taken by a professional on behalf of self or another may harm a third party, one toward whom the professional also has a duty of some kind. Ideally, then, conflict-of-interest rules minimize or eliminate risk of harm. Unfortunately, separating risk of harm from harm itself is not an easy task when creating and enforcing rules. This is a problem shared by all professional groups. Because economic incentives often create conflict-of-interest situations for professionals, the term *financial conflict of interest* has become the key to understanding the main problems (and proposed solutions) in biomedical research. That term is not prominent in the literature on conflict of interest for lawyers, although conflicting economic incentives are also a core problem for lawyers. This chapter attempts to explain how lawyers have struggled to articulate and solve conflict-of-interest problems. As has happened for their counterparts in biomedical research, lawyers' changing understanding of their societal roles has added another dimension to this complicated effort.

Lawyers represent clients, are officers in a complex legal system, and are public citizens, with special responsibility to justice. So says the preamble to the American Bar Association's (ABA) Model Rules of Professional Conduct of 1983,[1] which contains the rules that spell out the way in which these various roles are to be performed by lawyers in practice. The preamble continues:

> A lawyer's responsibilities as a representative of clients, an officer of the legal system and a public citizen are usually harmonious . . . In the nature of law practice, however, conflicting responsibilities are encountered. Virtually all

difficult ethical problems arise from conflict between a lawyer's responsibilities to clients, to the legal system and to the lawyer's own interest in remaining an ethical person while earning a satisfactory living.

The conflict of roles expressed in the preamble must be understood as necessary background to every rule contained in the Model Rules, including those specific conflict-of-interest rules with which this chapter is particularly concerned. Moreover, the manner in which the conflict-of-interest rules themselves have been understood and articulated has changed over time. Changed, as well, is the lawyer's understanding of the roles he or she plays. Indeed, the lawyer's understanding of the very nature of a profession has also changed. Most of these changes have been gradual and, some, controversial. Lawyers' acceptance of these changes has varied. As rules and enforceable, they cannot be denied. As principles of ethics, they may or may not represent the standards of the profession. What also cannot be denied is that the current milieu in which law practice is conducted is highly competitive in a way that lawyers in previous generations would not have been able to comprehend. Many of the specific conflict-of-interest rules and the current problems surrounding those rules are directly related to that accelerated and accelerating competition. To understand lawyers' conflict of interest in today's world, it is necessary to first acquire some historical perspective.

A Bit of History

Although lawyers have recognized conflicting interests as an ethics problem since the beginnings of the English Bar (Wolfram 1986) and the effort to refine the nature of the problem continues, the current conflict-of-interest rules do not comprise a unified set with anything like a unified theory undergirding them. Looking only at the American Bar's attempt to define and refine conflicts doctrine in the twentieth century, we find that the first major code of ethics, the Canons of Professional Ethics,[2] promulgated by the then fledgling ABA in 1908, contained three, largely hortatory paragraphs that did little more than identify a range of issues. Canon 6, entitled "Adverse Influences and Conflicting Interests," reads as follows:

It is the duty of the lawyer at the time of retainer to disclose to the client all the circumstances of his relation to the parties, and any interest in or connection with the controversy, which might influence the client in the selection of counsel.

It is unprofessional to represent conflicting interests, except by express consent of all concerned given after a full disclosure of the facts. Within the meaning of this canon, a lawyer represents conflicting interests when, in behalf of one client, it is his duty to contend for that which duty to another client requires him to oppose.

The obligation to represent the client with undivided fidelity and not to divulge his secrets or confidences forbids also the subsequent acceptance of retainers or employment from others in matters adversely affecting any interest of the client with respect to which confidence has been reposed.

The first paragraph and the first sentence of the second paragraph speak to what is really one kind of remedy for one kind of conflict of interest (what today we would call informed consent in concurrent-representation cases). The rest of paragraph two represents a stab at a definition but is instead only one example of one kind of conflict. The third paragraph identifies two of the major policy concerns of all conflicts doctrine (client loyalty and confidentiality), but it also references what is today called the subsequent-representation issue, which has always been treated differently from the concurrent-representation issue, although the concurrent-representation issue is implied as the central conflicts problem in the rest of canon 6. Thus, many of the issues of conflict of interest that plague the American Bar today were at least recognized as long ago as 1908, but the articulation of the conflicts and of the appropriate remedies for a variety of conflicts problems was woefully inadequate. This was due not only to a lack of a unifying theory of conflict of interest but also to the structure of the Canons of Ethics: mostly hortatory paragraphs like those found in canon 6. Moreover, the original thirty-two canons were not coherently organized. There was no reason why one particular canon followed another.

Because the locus for admitting lawyers to the bar and for sanctioning them lies with each jurisdiction, the states had to pass their own versions of the Canons of Ethics, which they quickly did. Although fifteen amendments were enacted in the intervening years, not until 1969 was the Canons of Ethics completely overhauled, with the passage by the ABA of the Model Code of Professional Responsibility.[3] The Model Code was divided into three parts: (1) a general "Canon" (nine new canons in all), which largely identified the basic principle to be addressed; (2) a series of "Ethical Considerations," which were to be aspirational in nature; and (3) a number of black-letter "Disciplinary Rules" (clear and binding norms), which set minimum standards below which no lawyer should fall, lest he or she risk formal sanction.

Conflict-of-interest rules and aspirations were largely contained in new canon 5, which read: "A Lawyer Should Exercise Independent Professional Judgment on Behalf of a Client." What followed was a series of twenty-four ethical considerations and six disciplinary rules (DR), each containing multiple subrules. The basic rules were contained in DR 5-105, which forbade a lawyer to accept or continue employment "if the Interests of Another Client May Impair the Independent Professional Judgment of the Lawyer." DR 5-105(A) and DR 5-105(B) forbade accepting or continuing employment if the lawyer's independent professional judgment "will be or is likely to be adversely affected" by representing another client. In addition, the Model Code was amended in 1974 to also prohibit representation "if it would be likely to involve" the lawyer "in representing differing interests." The term *differing interests* was defined as including "every interest that will adversely affect either the judgment or the loyalty of a lawyer to a client, whether it be a conflicting, inconsistent, diverse or other interest." Many states did not adopt the "differing interests" language, but it hardly mattered much, because there was no perceptible difference in results throughout the states whether the amendment was passed or not (Wolfram 1986). Presumably this was so because the traditional concept of "conflicting interests," which was inartfully expressed in the 1908 Canons of Ethics, already translated into something like a concern that a lawyer's independent professional judgment must remain unclouded. Clearly, "client loyalty" in concurrent-representation cases was already a bedrock principle, and the use of phrases such as "any interest" and "all the circumstances" suggested lawyers' broad range of concerns with any kind of potentially compromising interest.

With the Model Code, a theory of conflict of interest began to emerge. Lawyers were to refuse or discontinue work for a client if the lawyer's independent professional judgment would be or was "likely" to be impaired by work for another client. Presumably this formulation was clearer and more concrete than the language of canon 6 in the 1908 Canons of Ethics. New canon 5 in the Model Code, however, went much farther than the 1908 Canons and addressed several other specific conflict-of-interest issues. Although the specific issues might also have been seen as potential compromises to independent judgment, they were not always addressed that way. DR 5-101 did adopt the language of "independent professional judgment" and stated that the lawyer should not accept employment if professional judgment might be affected "by his own financial, business, property, or personal interest." Thus, it was not just another client's interest that might impair a lawyer's judgment but the lawyer's own interests as well. Moreover, these interests were not limited to "financial" conflicts but were broadly defined. Independent judgment may have been implied, but it was unstated in DR 5-101(B), which disallowed the lawyer or law firm to act as a witness. DR 5-102 dealt with the withdrawal of the lawyer or law firm after representation had begun. DR 5-103 specifically prohibited a lawyer from acquiring an interest in litigation. DR 5-104 limited business relations with the client. DR 5-106 forbade the lawyer to settle similar claims of clients. Finally, DR 5-107 set forth elaborate provisions regarding "Avoiding Influence by Others Than the Client." In each of these disciplinary rules, exceptions were specifically provided. Moreover, most of the rules also allowed representation by the lawyer with the informed consent of the client or clients.

Why the drafters did not do a better job in grouping the rules to reflect at least the emerging underlying theory (i.e., the risk to professional judgment posed by other "interests") is not altogether clear. Perhaps they did not do so because they did not believe there was a consistent underlying theory. In addition, specific rules about conflicts had begun to emerge in actual cases, and the drafters wanted to use those legal rules to establish a baseline for lawyer's discipline. In any event, the question of what was permitted under law began to be inexorably mixed with the ethical rules, which were not originally intended to solve concrete issues in litigation or in other legal contexts. Instead, they were supposed to (1) set a higher standard for all lawyers as a guide to good professional behavior, and (2) provide minimum standards to help police the profession. What was good for handling disputes for the general society might not be best for keeping lawyers functioning at a high ethical level. But the idea that ethics rules should be legal rules won the day when the ABA passed yet another ethics code in 1983—the Model Rules of Professional Conduct. The adoption of the Model Rules came a scant fourteen years after passage of the Model Code. Adoption of the Model Rules was a slow process in the states, and many of the specific rules were rejected. Uniformity is still an issue across jurisdictions, even though every state except California now uses the Model Rules format and much of its text as its basic pattern (ABA/BNA Lawyers' Manual on Professional Conduct 2009, 1:3–6).[4] The original Canons of Ethics, on the other hand, had lasted sixty-one years before its demise at the hands of the Model Code. It had also stayed relatively uniform across jurisdictions.

Rapid changes ensued across the ethics landscape, even as the Model Rules of Professional Conduct was sold to the practicing bar as "law for lawyers" (Patterson 1977). Law had trumped ethics rules as guidelines for ethical behavior. The original professional ideal was that codes of ethics were to be adopted by professional groups to set higher-than-ordinary ethical standards for the professional to use as a guide to behavior, thus assuring the public that members of the profession were eminently worthy of trust (Bayles 1981). The drafters' concern for promulgating clear and workable rules to discipline lawyers, however, distorted the way in which both the Model Code and the Model Rules were drafted. The change in titles alone, over the years, shows the nature of the problem. What was a set of Canons of Ethics became a Code of Professional Responsibility, which, in turn, became Rules of Professional Conduct. The very format of the Model Rules came from the American Law Institute's Restatements of Law: a black-letter rule, followed by commentary. Even the word *ethics* was all but banned from the document. The transformation from ethics to law was solidified in 1998 when, after a thirteen-year effort, the American Law Institute itself passed its Restatement of the Law Governing Lawyers (2000).[5] This restatement and the Model Rules share much in common: not only is the format identical, but the content is similar. The restatement attempts to set forth the rules most generally accepted as good law, taking all jurisdictions into account. The ABA's Model Rules is adapted and changed from state to state, and so are part of the restatement rules. The conflict-of-interest rules in the restatement are far more detailed than those in the ABA's Model Rules but follow them in essential ways.

Under basic disciplinary protocols, breaches of an ethics code may result in a private reprimand, a public reprimand, probation, suspension from practice, or disbarment (ABA/BNA Lawyer's Manual on Professional Conduct 2003, 101:3003). These four possible sanctions serve one goal only: not to punish lawyers, but to protect the public from unethical lawyers. Breaches of the law of lawyering, on the other hand, result in lawyers' disqualifications or monetary fines or in legal malpractice judgments. The underlying concern here is usually with the "fairness" of the trial between two litigants or compensation for particular, maltreated clients. Thus, ethical standards are primarily used by bar associations and state licensing bodies. They are of secondary importance to courts (ABA/BNA Lawyer's Manual on Professional

Conduct 2007, 51:1903). The Model Rules continues to state that the rules are not legal rules and should not be invoked for disqualification purposes or as "a basis for civil liability." Nevertheless, more and more lawyers (and judges) look to lawyers' ethics codes as enforceable legal rules (Report of the Commission on Professionalism 1986), not as descriptions of conduct that entails "obedience to the unforeseeable" (Drinker 1953). Earlier generations of lawyers conceived of ethical standards as designed to give aspirational guidance, not as providing rules to obey to keep their licenses.

To summarize: by the time of the passage of the Model Rules in 1983, three basic norms of professional conduct were implicated in conflict-of-interest rules. The first was the concept of client loyalty. At least with respect to a particular matter, the lawyer was to be the client's champion, not letting another client's interest or the lawyer's own self-interest compromise the lawyer's devotion. Second, in terms of doctrine, the lawyer's independent professional judgment was to be maintained against compromise. Third, client confidences, always of paramount important in a lawyer's hierarchy of values, were to be especially protected from disclosure, even after the lawyer-client relationship was terminated. Most of these values were protected by rather rigid rules, prophylactic in the main, which protected these client-centered values without much delving into facts. Even exceptions for, say, client consent were drafted in ways that did not allow lawyers much leeway in accepting cases that could compromise these values.

Nevertheless, the winds of change were blowing. As lawyers became more explicit economic actors, affiliating and disaffiliating with firms for perceived economic or other advantages, courts began to shape conflicts rules to fit this new reality. New rules were adopted to keep litigation moving ahead without being sidetracked by disputes over disqualifications of lawyers because of alleged conflicts of interest. These new rules were then taken into the 1983 Model Rules, without much concern that rules made for the practical purpose of moving litigation forward were not necessarily useful in determining how lawyers, pledged to a higher standard of ethics, should conduct themselves beforehand.

The Model Rules

In the rest of this chapter, I attempt to describe and critique the conflict-of-interest provisions of the Model Rules of Professional Conduct, as amended to February 2009. The preceding historical sketch identified two interlocking problems and hinted at a third. The first problem is the lack of a unified theory of conflict of interest. The second is the substantive rules themselves, as a confusing mix of law and ethics. The third problem emerges directly from the second: what is to be done when a conflict is identified? As we shall see, because lawyers' mobility is on the increase, and because it is generally believed to be a good thing that clients should be able to choose their own lawyers (and lawyers, their clients), remedies for managing conflicts are on the increase. Let us take up the theoretical problem first.

Toward a Theory of Lawyers' Conflict of Interest

Kevin McMunigal (2001) articulated a theory of conflict of interest that critiques conflicts doctrine as failing clearly "to recognize conflict of interest as a type of risk analysis aimed at setting acceptable risk levels regarding perverse incentives." Every lawyer (indeed, every professional, perhaps every ordinary person) sometimes has an incentive to do X for A, when X would not be optimal for B, and A and B are each people or groups that the lawyer has either a duty or an interest in protecting or benefiting. Michael Davis (2001) thinks this description is too broad and instead puts forth what he calls the "standard view" of all conflict of interest, which seems to be directly connected to the view that began to emerge in the Code of Professional Responsibility (i.e., a risk that the lawyer's independent professional judgment for a client may be compromised by another interest). Briefly, Davis's articulation of the "standard view" is this: "A conflict of interest is a situation in which some person P (whether an individual or corporate body) stands in a certain relation to one or more decisions. On the standard view, P has a conflict of interest if, and only if, (1) P is in a relationship with another requiring P to exercise judgment in the other's behalf and (2) P has a (special) interest tending to interfere with the proper exercise of judgment in that relationship" (Davis 2001).

Despite significant differences in the views held by McMunigal and Davis, they both see conflict of interest as a problem of "risk of harm," not harm itself. Davis thinks "professional judgment" (a key and a limiting term) is the value being protected by these rules, while McMunigal speaks of protecting "professional duties" (a broader term). I side with McMunigal, because the conflict does not always have an effect on the lawyer's professional judgment, as Davis uses that term. (According to Davis, a professional judgment is a decision needing "knowledge, skill, and insight to bear in unpredictable ways.")

Sometimes, a conflict of interest risks pushing the lawyer away from performing what may be a routine duty (i.e., one that does not require professional judgment but is obviously the right thing to do). A good example is the duty not to steal from a client. In any event, although the debate between the two scholars is interesting, it need not trouble us further. It is clear that the Model Rules does not embrace Davis's "standard view," even as it does not fully adopt McMunigal's analysis. Under either view, risk, not actual harm, is the issue.

Therefore, one problem with the Model Rules is that it mixes risk rules and harm rules. This problem is further compounded because the general "risk" rule is not identified as general, and there is a plethora of rules identified as conflict-of-interest rules, some of which are really "harm" rules. Before citing examples, let us be clear about the difference between risk and harm. A harm rule directly forbids a substantive wrong. For example, under model rule (MR) 7.3(b)(2), lawyers may not use coercion, duress, or harassment when soliciting potential clients. Contrariwise, a risk rule insulates the lawyer from a situation where a substantive wrong may occur. For example, under MR 7.3(a), a lawyer may not engage in personal solicitation for pecuniary gain—this avoids a situation where coercion, duress, or harassment may take place.

When it comes to conflict-of-interest rules themselves, McMunigal (2001) cites MR 1.8(a) as a classic case where risk and harm are mixed. The rule forbids a lawyer entering into a business transaction with a client ("clearly a high-risk situation") unless the terms are substantively "fair and reasonable to the client." ("This is a harm rule.")

One of the reasons conflict-of-interest rules are often dismissed as silly or merely technical is the lack of appreciation of the risk of harm that is often at the heart of the matter. As long as the person believes he or she has done no real harm, he or she is unwilling to admit the value of the rule. This may lead even well-meaning people to cross lines without noticing. For a refreshing self-analysis of the nature of the problem, see the article by psychiatrist Daniel Carlat (2007) entitled "Dr. Drug Rep." Dr. Carlat was paid handsomely by a drug company to talk with other doctors about the use of a certain drug he himself prescribed. The article details how Carlat excused or suppressed negative information about the drug, until he finally realized that his own professional judgment and personal honesty had been compromised. A rule forbidding doctors who are being paid by drug or device companies talking to other doctors for the purpose of selling drugs or devices would be a valuable conflicts rule. It would be like the rule that bars doctors from owning labs to which they send patients for tests. Both situations represent classic cases in which it is hard to demonstrate harm, because of the subtleties of judgment, but easy to see the risk of harm. This is as true for lawyers as it is for doctors.

Drafting conflict-of-interest rules as "risk" rules is only a first step. As Carlat's story suggests, there is an even deeper problem: what to do about a conflict of interest once it is identified. Increasingly, lawyers' conflicts rules are drafted so that they may be avoided or evaded. It is also the case that lawyers are rarely, if ever, disciplined for breaching conflict-of-interest rules, so, increasingly, conflict-of-interest case law (or practice realities) determines the substance of the rules. Moreover, even when legal rules do not become part of the Model Rules, the drafting of remedies tends to be more like black-letter law. To understand better what is happening, we need to look at the substantive rules and their remedies together. Davis describes three categories of remedy. The first, "escape," which used to be preferred by the drafters of lawyers' codes of ethics, means simply that the lawyer is not permitted to proceed with the work in question. The second category is "disclosure," which means disclosure to the client or clients, sometimes followed by the consent of the affected clients, although consent is not always necessary. Finally, the third category is "managing." Although Davis suggests that this category is often used with disclosure, he takes pains to show that this is not necessarily so. Increasingly, "managing" a conflict means just that—taking some care to avoid impairment, often by adding layers of protection or by partially realigning interests. The Model Rules uses disclosure and managing much more than escape.

Rules and Remedies
CURRENT CLIENTS

The Canons of Professional Ethics was most concerned with conflicts of interest between or among two or more clients or potential clients of the same lawyer. Although conflicts among current clients no longer dominate the conflicts landscape as they did in 1908, conflicts affecting "current clients" still occupy a central place in the Model Rules and illustrate the basic, general rule (see box). Recall the Model Code's central concern: the risk that the lawyer's independent professional judgment would be impaired by another interest. The Model Code used differing triggering standards to identify what was an unacceptable risk. If a second client's interests were involved, the words used were: "will be or is likely to be adversely affected." If the lawyer's own interests were involved, the words used were: "will be or reasonably may be affected." The difference between "likely to be adversely affected" and "reasonably may be affected" is unclear and perhaps unimportant. Recall, too, that when dealing with concurrent clients, the 1974 amendment to the Model Code prohibited representation "if it would be likely to involve" the lawyer "in representing differing interests." "Differing interests" was then broadly defined.

Contrast the language of the Model Code with that of the Model Rules. MR 1.7 is the basic rule on current clients, comparable to DR 5-105 and DR 5-101 quoted above. MR 1.7(a) prohibits representation if: "(1) the representation of one client will be directly adverse to another client; or (2) there is a significant risk that the representation of one or more clients will be materially limited by the lawyer's responsibilities to another client, a former client or a third person or by a personal interest of the lawyer." The two rules replicate the two categories identified in the Model Code (representing differing interests and the risk of impairment to judgment), but the substantive rules read differently.

MR 1.7(a)(1) eliminates concerns about a wide variety of "differing interests" and substitutes a prohibition simply on representing interests that are "directly adverse." MR 1.7(a)(2) adopts the language of "risk," modifying it by use of the word "significant" and substituting the qualifying "materially limited" by any other responsibility the lawyer has to another or to the lawyer's own interest. This seems to reinstate the meaning of "differing interests" by using concrete examples. Commentators tend to assume that the substance of MR 1.7(a)(1) and (a)(2) is the same as that of DR 5-105(a) and (b) and DR 5-101(a), but believe that the language is clearer, more precise, and therefore more helpful in the Model Rules. Maybe. Clearly, the Model Rules provides more wiggle room for lawyers to become involved in situations where their independent judgment on behalf of one client may be compromised by representation of a second client or by the lawyer's own interests directly.

Yet the paradigm cases surely come out the same way under the Model Code or the Model Rules. Because loyalty is the key value in current-client situations, without informed consent, a lawyer could never represent client A in any matter "directly adverse" to client B in any matter whatsoever, regardless of its lack of connection with the matter concerning client A. Why this concern could not be expressed in terms of "risk" is answered only by history. The prohibition against representing "differing interests" was added to the Model Code, even though the likelihood of impairment to a lawyer's independent professional judgment seemed to hold for situations covered by the language of "differing interests." Some lawyers just seemed to be more comfortable with the additional language.

There is an additional practical problem for lawyers working in firms. If lawyer A is disqualified from representing both X and Y in case 1, where X and Y are on opposite sides of the dispute, and both X and Y are current clients, then all the lawyers practicing with A are also disqualified. This is covered by MR 1.10(a) and DR 5-105(d). The reason behind such imputed disqualification is that lawyers in a single economic unit might favor one client over another in overt or covert ways. They may also breach confidentiality directly or carelessly. Because loyalty is the key factor here, the lawyer pledges not only his or her own loyalty and care but also that of all who work in the same law firm.

The case of *IBM v. Levin* (579 F.2d 271 [3d Cir. 1978]) is a good example of how scrupulously this prohibition was enforced by traditional courts. From 1970 to 1972, the CBM law firm represented IBM in four separate labor law matters. In 1972, CBM filed an antitrust suit against IBM on behalf of another client. At the time of the filing of the antitrust suit, CBM was not engaged in doing any legal work for IBM. Subsequently, however, CBM did represent IBM in four more labor law matters, until, in 1977, IBM filed a motion for disqualification of CBM in the antitrust case. The motion was granted. Although the trial court found as a fact that the in-house IBM lawyers working on the antitrust case were ignorant of the fact that other in-house lawyers were retaining CBM to work on labor matters for IBM until 1977, and no actual impairment to judgment or to duty was shown, nevertheless, the risk of harm was considered real and intolerable in situations where a firm both sues and defends the same party, even in disparate cases. This case shows that the issue of risk is relevant even when the facts demonstrate "directly adverse" representation. The court in *Levin* used the Model Code provision on "independent professional judgment" as the crucial norm. The "differing interests" language was not adopted in the relevant jurisdiction at the time. Today, the case should come out the same way; either MR 1.7(a)(1) or MR 1.7(a)(2) would suffice to do the job. However, issues of consent increasingly muddy the waters.

In the *Levin* case, the plaintiffs argued that IBM had consented to the multiple concurrent representations. The court dismissed the argument by saying that, under the facts, there had not been sufficient explanation on the part of the CBM lawyers as to the potential conflict, so true informed consent was not given. The implication was that proper informed consent might be given,

Current Clients: Specific Rules in the American Bar Association's Model Rules of Professional Conduct, 1983

MR 1.7 sets forth the basic, general rules regarding lawyers' conduct in relation to a current client. MR 1.8 sets forth a series of specific rules concerning the same relationship. Historically, many of these rules developed from case law, so it was natural for lawyers to incorporate them into their ethics codes, particularly as those codes began to look more law-like. Some direct antecedents to the present rules can be found in the 1908 Canons of Professional Ethics. For example, canon 10 stated that "the lawyer should not purchase any interest in the subject matter of litigation which he is conducting." And canon 19 simply stated that a lawyer should not be both a witness and an advocate in the same case. The 1969 Model Code of Professional Responsibility carried forth more elaborated versions of such rules—for example, in DR 5-102, dealing with the lawyer as witness, and in DR 5-103, which deals with the lawyer's not acquiring an interest in litigation. Although many of the present set of specific rules could, perhaps, be justified on the basis of a risk theory of conflict of interest, no attempt will be made to do so. Some rules clearly would not fit that theory. Instead, I indicate after each rule what important value seems to be at stake. What matters here is that the drafters of these rules thought each rule represented a conflict of interest in a current-client representation situation, so the rules need to be identified as such.

MR 1.8(a) forbids a lawyer from entering into a business transaction or relationship with a client unless the terms are "fair and reasonable to the client and are fully disclosed and transmitted . . . in a manner that can be reasonably understood." In addition, the client must be advised "in writing" of the usefulness of having independent counsel; and the client must give written informed consent. (Presumably, this protects clients from lawyers' taking advantage of them.)

MR 1.8(b) forbids the lawyer from using client information to the detriment of the client without informed consent. (This is a harm rule that protects against the misuse of client confidences.)

MR 1.8(c) forbids lawyers from receiving substantial gifts from clients and also prevents the lawyer from preparing any legal instrument that gives the lawyer or any of the lawyer's close relatives any substantial gifts. (This protects clients from lawyers' taking advantage of them.)

MR 1.8(d) forbids the lawyer from making or negotiating "an agreement giving the lawyer literary or media rights to a portrayal or account based in substantial part on information relating to the representation" of the client by the lawyer. The prohibition exists only until the representation ends. (This is designed to keep the lawyer from making a bad judgment for a client out of self-interest.)

MR 1.8(e) forbids the lawyer from providing "financial assistance" to a client in connection with litigation, except to an indigent client. The lawyer may advance "costs and expenses" of litigation to any other client, contingent on the outcome of the matter. (This is designed to prevent abuse of the legal system.)

MR 1.8(f) forbids a lawyer from accepting compensation from another person for representing a client, unless the client gives informed consent, confidentiality is protected, and "there is no interference with the lawyer's professional judgment or with the lawyer-client relationship." (This is to keep client loyalty foremost in the lawyer's representative acts.)

MR 1.8(g) forbids the lawyer from making an agreement in any civil or criminal case settling a matter for two or more clients unless each gives informed consent. (This ensures that no client is compromised for another.)

MR 1.8(h) forbids the lawyer from making an agreement "prospectively limiting the lawyer's liability to a client for malpractice unless the client is independently represented." It also forbids the lawyer from settling claims for malpractice with a client or former client unless each is advised of the "desirability of seeking and is given a reasonable opportunity to seek the advice" of another independent lawyer. (This prevents lawyers' taking advantage of clients.)

MR 1.8(i) forbids the lawyer from acquiring a "proprietary interest" in litigation, except "a lien authorized by law" or under a contingent fee arrangement. (This is designed to prevent abuse of the legal system.)

MR 1.8(j) forbids a lawyer from having a sexual relationship with a client "unless a consensual sexual relationship existed between them when the client-lawyer relationship commenced." (This is to prevent a lawyer's taking advantage of a client.)

MR 1.8(k) ensures that a lawyer disqualification under any provisions of MR 1.8 (except MR 1.8[j]) results in disqualification of all lawyers working with the disqualified lawyer. (This and other imputed disqualification rules are designed to prevent abuse of the system or client by persons working with the lawyer who is directly prohibited from doing something.)

at least in concurrent-representation cases such as *Levin*, where the subject matter of the work was sufficiently disparate. However, under the Model Code, the uses of informed consent were governed by a strict rule. Again, this seemed to offer added protection to clients. Under DR 5-105(c), a lawyer (or a law firm) could represent multiple clients concurrently with informed consent, but only if it were also "obvious" that the lawyer or firm could "adequately represent the interest of each." The "obvious" test was a difficult hurdle to jump over. Indeed, the Oregon Supreme Court in *In re Porter* (584 P.2d 744, 749 n.5 [Oregon, 1978]) said that the word *obvious* makes "the representation of conflicting interests nearly impossible." When was it obvious that a lawyer's independent professional judgment would not be impaired by favoring one client over the other? The test was always based on a firm notion of client loyalty, and there was always a strong presumption that loyalty would be impaired by representing client A in any disputed situation with client B, where both A and B were clients.

Contrast the formulation under the Model Code with the one articulated in the current Model Rules. Under MR 1.7(b), the lawyer may represent clients with a conflict of interest concurrently if the clients give informed consent, if the lawyer (or law firm) "reasonably believes" that "competent and diligent representation" can be given to each client, if there is no prohibition under applicable law, and if "the representation does not involve the assertion of a claim by one client against another client represented by the lawyer in the same litigation or other proceeding before a tribunal." Because the "obvious" language of the Model Code has been deleted, it might be argued that the Model Rules has adopted a new standard, although some have argued that it has kept the same substantive rules, altering only the language for clarity. It is hard to read MR 1.7 as anything other than supplying a way to eliminate the risk associated with representing clients with a current conflict of interest, absent some evidence of impairment or favoritism existing at the time of the retainers. "Informed consent" seems to be a cure-all.

Because what we are talking about is subtle, perhaps undetectable impairment, as in Carlat's case discussed above, the professional ideal seems compromised. As a matter of law, perhaps the idea that "informed consent" can cure a conflict is a necessary rule. Or maybe this kind of rule ought to be established only for sophisticated clients. In fact, MR 1.7 is being widely read by bar associations' committees on ethics to mean that sophisticated clients not only can consent but also can consent in advance and without being fully informed beforehand. In an opinion by the Association of the Bar of the City of New York Committee on Professional and Judicial Ethics (Opinion No. 2006-1), the notion was advanced that client loyalty as traditionally understood was outdated. The reasons given were twofold. First, "the market for legal services had changed drastically" over the years. Clients now hired multiple law firms, thus diminishing loyalty on both sides and greatly increasing the number of potential conflicts. And second, "the resulting increase in the number of potential lawyer-client conflicts has been accompanied by an increase in tactical disqualification motions." Although the emphasis was on the changes in the legal services market for large law firms, the opinion also said that an "overly broad interpretation of the duty of loyalty also visits significant injury on law firms of all sizes." Comment 22 to MR 1.7 explicitly endorsed the view that advance-consent waivers were now acceptable under the Model Rules; and in 2005, the ABA Standing Committee on Ethics and Professional Responsibility (Formal Opinion 05-436) conceded that MR 1.7, as amended in 2002, "permits effective informed consent to a wider range of future conflicts than would have been possible under the Model Rules prior to their amendment." It may be that unsophisticated clients also are permitted to consent, although their lawyers may be bound to explain the potential problems of consenting to this conflict of interest with more clarity and in greater detail. Presumably, increased competition among lawyers is a driving force behind the loosening of the basic current-client rule.

My point is not to condemn the effort to make the legal rules more nuanced as the world changes. It is to demonstrate that law and ethics are becoming inextricably connected and that the details of conflict-of-interest law are becoming increasingly difficult to apply in more and more cases. Nowhere is this seen more clearly than in the cases involving former clients, the so-called subsequent-representation cases, governed by MR 1.9.

FORMER CLIENTS

Loyalty issues diminish as lawyers and clients part ways, as loyalty "is the willing . . . and thorough going devotion of a person to a cause" (J. Royce, "The Philosophy of Loyalty" [1908], quoted in Lawry 1990, 1102). Thus, all that remains of loyalty after the engagement has been terminated is whatever has resulted from the work performed. Thus, it would certainly be professionally inappropriate for a lawyer to upset a will that he or she had previously drafted for a former client. However, one other professional obligation also remains: the obligation to keep client confidences in perpetuity. The prohibition against disclosing confidences of former clients was identified in canon 6 of the 1908 Canons of Ethics and is now generally incorporated in MR 1.6 and in MR 1.9(c) of the Model Rules. An additional independent conflict-of-interest rule, guarding against the risk of such impermissible disclosures, was first announced in 1953 in *T.C. Theatre Corp v. Warner Bros. Pictures* (113 F. Supp. 265, 268–269 [S.D.N.Y. 1953]). In this case, Judge Weinfeld established the "substantial relationship test," described as follows:

> The former client need show no more than [that] the matters embraced within the pending suit wherein his former attorney appears on behalf of his adversary are substantially related to the matters or the cause of action wherein the attorney previously represented him, the former client. The Court will assume that during the course of the former representation confidences were disclosed to the attorney bearing on the subject matter of the representation.

This test is currently incorporated in MR 1.9(a) of the Model Rules and simply avoids the risk of disclosure of confidential information by preventing the lawyer from representing another client in any matter "substantially related" to a prior representation for a former client. As it stands, MR 1.9(a) seems prophylactic and would, of course, be imputed to the lawyer's law firm as well, under MR 1.10. However, it is here that a relatively new question has arisen: screening. The concept is defined under MR 1.0(k) as follows:

> "Screened" denotes the isolation of a lawyer from any participation in a matter through the timely imposition of procedures within a firm that are reasonably adequate under the circumstances to protect information that the isolated lawyer is obligated to protect under these rules or other law.

Although screens had been used by accounting firms to isolate the attest function from other work, most lawyers were introduced to the idea in 1975 by the ABA Standing Committee on Ethics, in Formal Opinion 342. The opinion argued that unless former government lawyers were permitted to be screened, and the firms they joined were permitted to represent clients in situations barred by the usual imputed disqualification rule, good lawyers would avoid government work, to the detriment of the common good. This opinion was handed down in the teeth of clear language to the contrary in the then almost universally adopted Model Code. Case law began to follow the ABA opinion, and MR 1.11(b) explicitly allowed such screening for former government lawyers—but not for private lawyers moving from firm to firm. Initially, the Model Rules made no change in the prohibition against the use of screens in cases involving the movement of nongovernment lawyers. As we shall see, that prohibition was recently lifted by the ABA.

Although courts were historically reluctant to allow screening in private lawyers' cases, that reluctance is giving way because private law firms are using screens so frequently that the behavior of the bar seems to have completely reversed the prohibition against screens in nongovernment cases, too—at least in some jurisdictions. According to the most recent statistics on the matter, some twenty-three of fifty-one jurisdictions allow at least limited screening without the consent of the former client (Morgan and Rotunda 2009, 169–74). The formal rule change often took place after there had been a judicial decision on the issue. This was true in Ohio, for example, where in *Kala v. Aluminum Smelting & Refining Co., Inc.* (81 Ohio St. 3d 1 [1998]), the state's Supreme Court indicated it would permit screening in cases where the lawyer would be disqualified because of the danger of disclosing confidential information from a former client, to that client's detriment. Screening would be disallowed only in cases in which the disqualified lawyers had substantial responsibility in the same matter itself. The actual ethics rule change occurred nine years later, in 2007, when Ohio finally adopted its own version of the Model Rules (Ohio Rules of Professional Conduct), indicating that the practice of the bar was to ignore the rule, presumably because lawyers' mobility was a reality that practicing lawyers felt they had to handle in a way that made the most pragmatic sense to them. It should be noted, however, that there are good arguments to support the older prohibition. Those arguments are based on the risk of disclosure to aid the new client or of an inadvertent breach, given that screens are created by fallible human beings. At the end of the day, it is clear that many lawyers are sometimes disobeying even clear ethics rules pertaining to conflicts of interest, then challenging those rules in courts—concerned only about what the courts will do and letting the ethics rules change later, but unconcerned about whether they change at all. This is a worrisome trend.

In February 2009, the ABA made a radical change in the screening rules, governing situations where a lawyer moves from one firm to another. Under new MR 1.10(a)(2), no matter the extent of the prior representation of a former client or the confidential information the moving lawyer may possess, he or she may be screened without the former client's consent. All the new firm need do is take certain explicit steps to ensure the screen's workability, including reasonable responses to inquiries made by the former client. The debate on the issue was fierce. It was successfully argued that the increased mobility of both lawyers and clients required this change. The opposition's suggestion that the rule change was made "for the convenience of lawyers" and amounted to an assault on the basic professional values of "confidentiality and loyalty" was insufficient to stem the tide (ABA/BNA Lawyers' Manual 2009, 28:88). Currently, twenty-four states allow at least limited nonconsensual screening in private lawyers' cases, although only about a dozen go as far as the new ABA rule allows. It remains to be seen how many more states adopt this more radical amendment to the Model Rules.

MR 1.9(b) is another rule lifted directly from a case, *Silver Chrysler Plymouth, Inc. v. Chrysler Motors Corporation* (518 F.2d 751 [2d Circuit 1975]). The rule also deals with the situation where a lawyer moves from firm A to firm B. While the lawyer was with firm A, the firm represented client 1, in the same or a substantially related case, which is now the subject of a representation by firm B for client 2, which is "materially adverse" to client 1. Historically, because the moving lawyer would bring the application of the "substantially related" rule with him or her when changing firms, both the lawyer and the new firm would be disqualified. Under MR 1.9 and MR 1.10, that would still be the case generally (unless some special screening rule, as discussed above, were in place). But now, under MR 1.9(b), the moving lawyer does not bring the taint (of knowing confidential information) with him or her, as long as it can be shown that the lawyer did not acquire confidential information material to the new matter. Under the original "substantially related" test, it was assumed that the moving lawyer had such information by dint of his or her association with the first firm, with the result that both that lawyer and the new firm would be barred from representing client 2 against client 1 in the same or a substantially related matter. Now, the lawyer may represent client 2 against client 1 if, in an evidentiary hearing, it can be shown to the satisfaction of the judge that the lawyer had not acquired material confidential information. Of course, in those jurisdictions where a screening rule is allowed or simply generally practiced, it is often just easier to screen the incoming lawyer.

Most troublesome here is the difficulty that protesting firms encounter in trying to prove that the moving lawyer acquired such information. In the *Silver Chrysler* case, the moving lawyer seemed to have worked on substantially related matters, but the court said the work was merely technical and did not entail having to obtain important factual information. So, if the lawyer said he or she did not receive that kind of confidential information, it would be hard to prove otherwise. Even law partners deeply involved in the case may not know the extent of the information the lawyer obtained. Here, lawyers' mobility was cited as an important factor in deciding the case—and thus in loosening the conflicts rule.

The new rules dealing with former clients represent the clearest indication that conflict-of-interest rules are now being adopted with more concern for the plight of lawyers in a competitive market than for strong assurances that client confidences will be maintained. Screening is the example *par excellence*. Critics suggest that the screen is easily penetrated with no reasonable ways for former clients to detect breaches. The original drafters of the Model Rules agreed; but the 2009 amendment to MR 1.10 finds the problem less troublesome. The history on this issue is clear. Firms began to defy the rules. Courts then followed the lead of the lawyers. And the ethics rules followed the changes that courts were making. Over the past twenty-five years or more, the idea that ethics rules should actually be "law for lawyers" has slowly taken hold in the United States. How to prevent law from undermining basic ethics principles has become the major twenty-first century problem for lawyers. Law usually represents a minimum standard, adopted for practical reasons. Professional ethics has traditionally been about norms above the minimum, as a pledge by a specialized group to serve selflessly the needs of those who may not easily know what the practitioner is about. Concerns about the deprofessionalization of lawyers thus abound.

Conclusion

The conflict-of-interest rules governing lawyers are a complex set of detailed prohibitions, often accompanied by significant exceptions. Because mobility has become such an important part of modern law practice, the rules have changed to more often allow lawyers to represent clients despite a conflict of interest. Most of the changes have taken place as a direct result of case-law decisions, where pragmatic factors often overcome real risks that lawyers may harm current or former clients. These kinds of legal rules, which set minimum standards in particular factual circumstances, now trump broader ethical norms, which should give high-level guidance to good practice. Thus, conflict-of-interest rules have weakened over time.

The trend in legal practice toward allowing more self-management of conflicts mirrors the trend in biomedical research. Simply allowing informed consent of clients to cure conflicts often obscures the fact that it is difficult to see clearly into the future or to appreciate the extent of the pressure to compromise professional standards that those in a conflict situation may feel. Screening without former client consent is an even more troubling fact of modern law practice. Both current trends seem to minimize the public service dimension of legal practice. This does not bode well for the continued self-regulation of the legal profession, an issue not discussed in this chapter, but one that should concern lawyers as a professional group and all citizens.

NOTES

1. This document is hereafter referred to simply as the Model Rules (available in its most recently amended form at www.abanet.org/cpr).

2. Hereafter referred to as the Canons of Ethics (www.abanet.org/cpr).

3. Hereafter referred to as the Model Code (www.abanet.org/cpr).

4. ABA/BNA Lawyer's Manual on Professional Conduct (Chicago: American Bar Association and Bureau of National Affairs, various years).

5. American Law Institute, "Restatement of the Law," 3rd Restatement, The Law Governing Lawyers (2000).

REFERENCES

Bayles, M. 1981. *Professional Ethics*. Belmont, CA: Wadsworth.
Carlat, D. 2007. Dr. Drug Rep. *New York Times Magazine*, Nov. 25.
Davis, M. 2001. Introduction. In *Conflict of Interest in the Professions*, ed. M. Davis and A. Stark, 3–19. New York: Oxford University Press.
Davis, M., and A. Stark, eds. 2001. *Conflict of Interest in the Professions*. New York: Oxford University Press.
Drinker, H. 1953. *Legal Ethics*. New York: Columbia University Press.
Lawry, R. 1990. The meaning of loyalty. *Capital University Law Review* 19:1089–1116.
McMunigal, K. 2001. Conflict of interest as risk analysis. In *Conflict of Interest in the Professions*, ed. M. Davis and A. Stark, 61–70. New York: Oxford University Press.
Morgan, T. D., and D. Rotunda. 2008. *Selected Standards on Professional Responsibility*. New York: Foundation Press.
Patterson, E. 1977. Wanted: A new code of professional responsibility. *ABA Journal* 63:639–42.
Report of the Commission on Professionalism to the Board of Governors and the House of Delegates of the American Bar Association. 1986. ". . . In the Spirit of Public Service": A Blueprint for the Rekindling of Lawyer Professionalism. *Federal Rules Decisions* 112:243–321.
Wolfram, C. W. 1986. *Modern Legal Ethics*. St. Paul, MN: West Publishing.

CHAPTER 7

Sustaining Credibility in a Context of Conflicts

The Challenge for Journalism

DENI ELLIOTT, PH.D.

Television news reporter Mirthala Salinas announced to the Los Angeles Telemundo viewers on June 8, 2007, that Los Angeles Mayor Antonio Villaraigosa and his wife of 20 years were separating. She didn't disclose a material fact that she knew: this marriage was dissolving because the mayor had been having an affair. She also didn't disclose that she was the woman with whom he was having the affair. By early July, both the mayor and the reporter had publicly confirmed that they were romantically involved. Salinas was first placed on administrative leave. After a month-long internal investigation by her employer, she received a two-month suspension for violation of the station's conflict-of-interest policies, for both her involvement with the mayor and her failure to disclose the relationship to her employers. Upon returning to work, Salinas was reassigned from Los Angeles to Riverside County, and she resigned.

This is the conventional journalistic conflict-of-interest story. A journalist gets too cozy with her source and is disciplined. But the problem of conflicting desires or loyalties in journalism is more complex than the need for reporters to refrain from having sex with their sources. Far more interesting are the subtle conflicts of interest and conflicts of commitment that individual journalists face but rarely acknowledge. Far more intriguing are the institutional conflicts of interest and conflicts of commitment that are almost never labeled as such. These conflicts can threaten the credibility of journalists and the news organizations for which they work. Journalists have long prized their independence and ability to report the truth fairly and accurately, which is why journalism has developed strong stances on conflicts of interest and conflicts of commitment. However, as in other professions, these stances risk being undermined by changes in structure and funding.

This chapter describes the scope of conflicts that impede, or can be perceived as impeding, journalists in doing their jobs and explains why the mere appearance of a conflict of interest matters to journalists and their news-organization employers. It reviews some individual conflicts and organizational conflicts and explains why those conflicts are of concern to journalism and what is being done to address them. It also considers how the expansion of reporting platforms to include the web and its cadre of citizen-journalists raises new questions for journalism and requires ongoing diligence.

The Job of Journalists

In a web-centric information era, journalists compete for public notice amid a cacophony of messages. For citizens to appropriately process journalistic messages, these must be distinguished from entertainment, public relations, advertising, and input from bloggers and the newly dubbed citizen-journalists. Traditionally, the role of journalist was first that of gatekeeper. There are many events and issues in the world that could be reported. Traditionally, what counted as "news," something worthy of a citizen's time and attention, was those issues and events chosen by editors and reporters. In the twentieth century, if a news organization did not report on an issue or event, it went largely unnoticed. By the start of the twenty-first century, anyone with access to a computer or a cell phone with a camera could, in turn, be a news producer and consumer. Members of the public can access information without relying on journalists to provide it.

The journalist's traditional role as gatekeeper and primary channel of information to citizens has certainly diminished, but, ironically, the social institution of journalism is more important than ever. The special role-related responsibility of journalism now, as before, is to provide citizens with information we need for self-governance. The essential shared value of journalism, which distinguishes that practice from other media and other information-givers, is that of timely truth-telling. In the midst of a virtual world of message-givers, journalists must make efforts to ensure that audience members recognize them as credible information sources that provide the reliable evidence necessary for audience members to be educated decision makers in a democracy. According to media ethics scholars Sandra Borden and Michael Pritchard (2001, 75), "Journalists, however else they might be characterized, have responsibilities grounded in their protected social function of gathering, interpreting, presenting, and disseminating information needed for individuals and communities to make sound judgments about matters of personal, political, and social importance."

Research shows that working journalists know where their primary loyalty should lie. In a 1999 survey on values by the Pew Research Center for the People and the Press and the Committee of Concerned Journalists, more than 80 percent of respondents listed "making the reader/listener/viewer your first obligation" as a "core principle of journalism." In separate open-ended, in-depth interviews with developmental psychologists, "more than 70 percent of journalists similarly placed 'audience' as their first loyalty, well above their employers, themselves, their profession, or even their families" (Kovach and Rosenstiel 2007, 53).

In contrast, as corporate ownership of news outlets has increased since the late twentieth century, the management of news has become firmly entrenched in a business model that seeks to produce the news "product" at the lowest cost and with maximum profit. The potential interorganizational conflict between making news and making money is ubiquitous. Traditionally, this issue was managed by the maintenance of a strict "wall" between the editorial function of a news organization (news gathering, reporting, and placement) and the business function (advertising and circulation). That wall has now eroded throughout the industry. According to Borden and Pritchard (2001, 88), "The solution of strictly demarcating editorial and business functions has been less effective as corporate linkages have become harder to disentangle and as management trends in journalism have begun to emphasize the integration of organizational functions." For example, Disney acquired the American Broadcasting Corporation (ABC), including ABC's news division, in 1996. Two years later, ABC pulled an investigative television news report on pedophiles working at Disney theme parks. While there is no consensus regarding the "real" reasons that the story did not run, the appearance of conflict of interest with the parent company is inescapable.

The Development of Dispassionate Journalism

The idea of the professional journalist who strives to serve the public interest in his or her reporting is a relatively new concept. As late as 1850, journalists moved between serving in political positions and reporting for partisan newspapers. In the early decades of the nineteenth century, "an editor generally berated the opposing party and leadership, so using any current measures of standards—such as accuracy or balance—is therefore irrelevant" (Dicken-Garcia 1989, 97). However, two forces were at work that gave rise to the development of the balanced, accurate, complete, and relevant (BARC) accounts that news organizations became known for in the twentieth century.

New presses and printing techniques allowed for cheap printing, which meant that newspapers were suddenly in the budget of all citizens, not just those with political power and agendas. Newspapers moved from filling a "political role" that served the needs of political parties or groups to an "information or news role" that provided "the individual with information useful in life's conduct, decision making, and participation in the political system." The editors who ran these cheap newspapers, dubbed the Penny Press, viewed "their role as fulfilling a duty to provide the news—not to serve a party or mercantile class; to provide a realistic view of contemporary life, despite taboos; to expose abuses wherever they were found; and to report items of human interest" (Dicken-Garcia 1989, 106–7). For the first time, U.S. news media were making enough money on their own and no longer needed to rely on the patronage of political parties.

In addition, the invention of the telegraph in the mid nineteenth century provided the impetus for the creation of the Associated Press, a wire service owned and shared by a cooperative of news organizations. News could be gathered far from the home newspaper and sent quickly through telegraph lines. Rather than each news organization bearing the expense of satellite bureaus and the cost of transmission, a collaborative pool of reporters and, later, photographers and then broadcast journalists could gather a story that was then distributed to all member organizations. This collaborative reporting required, then as now, a product that was suitable for a true "mass" audience, in which the news gatherers could make no assumptions about the political leanings or biases of the audience members. The goal of producing an "objective" news account was based on the idea of providing information that could be filtered through any reader's or viewer's political or personal biases. So, perhaps ironically, while reporting that serves no special interest other than accuracy is touted as an important ethical principle of journalism today, it rests on the technological and marketing values of the past. Through this notion of serving no special interest, the concern about conflicts of interest for journalists was born. By the late twentieth century, writers of media ethics textbooks assumed the importance of journalists' putting their professional obligations first.

Operational Definitions

Both individuals and institutions can have conflicts with external obligations and interests or within internal roles and expectations. Some of these are conflicts of interest; others are conflicts of commitment.

Conflicts of interest "are conflicts between professional interests and personal or financial interests. What distinguishes conflict of interest situations is that the conflict is between what one is trusted or expected to do in one's role . . . and financial or personal influences or interests that will or could compromise one's professional judgment and behavior in that role" (Werhane and Doering 1996, 51). A description of conflicts of interest as a prima facie wrong is typical in journalism textbooks: "When a reporter and editor no longer have a primary obligation or loyalty to their audiences but instead to someone else, problems of conflict of interest emerge" (Englehardt and Barney 1999, 181). Another author lists common examples of the kinds of financial interest that will generate conflicts of interest for journalists: "Junkets: expenses-paid trips that make it attractive for journalists to cover events . . . Freebies: gifts like free meals or tickets, to befriend or influence a media professional . . . Bribes: outright payments or promises to buy services or goods from a media outlet in return for some favor. For instance, a lawyer can promise to purchase advertising from a TV station if the station's general manager cancels an investigative consumer segment about a product manufactured by the lawyer's client" (Bugeja 2008, 198). The same author describes "nonmonetary conflicts" as follows:

> Personal vs. personal value: conflicts that occur when your personal value clashes with a personal value of a relative or other person outside your place of employment . . . Professional vs. professional value: conflicts that occur when one of your professional values directly conflicts with another of your professional values or when one of your professional values conflicts with a value of your co-worker, superior, client, source or employer. Personal vs. professional value: conflicts that occur when one of your personal values directly conflicts with one of your professional values or when one of your personal values conflicts with a professional value of your co-worker, superior, client, source or employer. (200)

Conflicts of commitment "are conflicts that entail a conflict between two or more sets of professional commitments that will affect one's focus of time, attention, and responsibility" (Werhane and Doering 1996, 51). Conflicts of commitment can also occur between personal and professional role commitments and between one's own professional commitment and one's commitment to a higher principle or external obligation.

All individuals and institutions face potentially conflicting situations. However, while conflicts of *interest* can be ethically managed through avoidance, recusal, or disclosure, conflicts of *commitment* may only sometimes be addressed in these ways. No one would wish to divest oneself of the various roles that most competent adults play—life partner, parent, child, friend, citizen, and volunteer—for one's professional role. Indeed, professional roles themselves inherently involve conflicts of commitment. Journalists are appropriately loyal to their professional peers and their employers, in addition to their primary loyalty to citizens. They may have too many stories to produce in too little time; they may need to compromise completeness in pursuit of a timely story. Thoughtful individuals and socially aware organizations live with the conscious awareness of the tension of competing obligations, sometimes deciding minute-by-minute which obligation has current priority.

The practice of journalism may be different from other professions in that nonmonetary conflicts, or conflicts of commitment, may be as troubling as financial conflicts. It is easy for most journalists to recognize the ethical problem inherent in someone offering them a bribe in exchange for killing a story. It is less clear for some reporters that failing to report material at the request of a friend or a loved one is just as much an ethical violation. Conflict-of-interest and conflict-of-commitment rules and expectations are based on the principle that any interest—financial or otherwise—that could deter a journalist from providing citizens with information they need requires attention.

Conflicts of Interest for Individual Journalists

Conflicts of interest for individuals can be obvious, such as a reporter having romantic or sexual interest in a source or a story subject or accepting a bribe to keep particular information out of a news story. These types of conflict could (and do) easily compromise an individual's ability to meet his or her professional obligations. Other common types of conflict of interest include outside employment, such as invitations to produce freelance work for a source, a potential source, or a competing news organization.

Most news organizations and professional news-gathering organizations provide guidelines recommending that journalists completely avoid at least some individual conflicts of interest. For example, the Society of Professional Journalists (1996) recommends to its members that "journalists should be free of obligation to any interest other than the public's right to know." Along with "avoiding conflicts of interest, real or perceived" and disclosing "unavoidable conflicts," members are counseled to "remain free of associations and activities that may compromise integrity or damage credibility," to "refuse gifts, favors, fees, free travel and special treatment, and shun secondary employment, political involvement, public office and service in community organizations if they compromise journalistic integrity," and to "deny favored treatment to advertisers and special interests and resist their pressure to influence news coverage."

After its eschewing codes of ethics for years, scandals in the early 2000s led the venerable New York Times to develop and publish a "policy" on ethics in journalism. The policy is based on the assumption that "the company, its separate business units and members of its newsrooms and editorial pages share an interest in avoiding conflicts of interest or any appearance of conflict." It notes that "conflicts of interest, real or apparent, may arise in many areas. They may involve tensions between journalists' professional obligations to our audience and their relationships with news sources, advocacy groups, advertisers, or competitors; with one another or with the company or one of its units. And at a time when two-career families are the norm, the civic and professional activities of spouses, household members and other relatives can create conflicts or the appearance of them." The Times warns those covered by the policy that "any intentional violation of these rules" is a serious offense "that may lead to disciplinary action, potentially including dismissal" (New York Times Company 2005). The fourteen-page document covers a variety of potentially conflicting situations and consistently makes the point that the company will not tolerate any behavior that might interfere with a journalist's neutrality or give the perception of interference, on or off the job.

Journalists who gather and produce images and sound are held to the same standard as their print counterparts. For example, the National Press Photographers Association's Code of Ethics (2006) says: "Do not accept gifts, favors, or compensation from those who might seek to influence coverage"; and, "Avoid political, civic and business involvements or other employment that compromise or give the appearance of compromising one's own journalistic independence." The Radio-Television News Directors Association and Foundation (2000) counsels its members to "understand that any commitment other than service to the public undermines trust and credibility," and not to "accept gifts, favors, or compensation from those who might seek to influence coverage" or "engage in activities that may compromise their integrity or independence." In addition, in a section labeled "Independence," members are issued the following reminder:

> Professional electronic journalists should: Gather and report news without fear or favor, and vigorously resist undue influence from any outside forces, including advertisers, sources, story subjects, powerful individuals, and special interest groups; Resist those who seek to buy or politically influence news content or who would seek to intimidate those who gather and disseminate the news; Determine news content solely through editorial judgment and not as the result of outside influence; Resist any self-interest or peer pressure that might erode journalistic duty and service to the public; Recognize that sponsorship of the news will not be used in any way to determine, restrict, or manipulate content; and Refuse to allow the interests of ownership or management to influence news judgment and content inappropriately.

The need to avoid interests that could interfere with the public interest is, therefore, a professional convention, regardless of the reporting platform.

When it comes to managing conflicts of interest, most news organizations, as is the case with the New York Times, prohibit newsroom employees from buying stock or engaging in financial transactions if there is a possibility that they had inside knowledge due to their journalistic status. Journalists are almost always prohibited from accepting compensation from any potential news source or story subject. Generally, they are not allowed to accept anything of value from anyone other than their employer, unless it is something that is offered to the general public. For example, journalists are generally allowed to accept frequent flyer miles for their personal or business-related trips but are not allowed to accept free flights from corporate sources. Exceptions may be made in military or government coverage, where there is no other way to get the story or no way to pay a travel fee.

Managing conflicts of interest when journalists do work on their own behalf, such as writing books or maintaining websites, is trickier. The material contained in a news story or production is usually a small portion of the information that the journalist collected. It is not unusual, therefore, for a journalist who has been involved in a long investigation or ongoing news story to be approached by an agent or publisher wishing to turn the journalist's observations and expertise into a book-length manuscript. Few news organizations have worked out, in advance, how to negotiate such interests. The New York Times disallows journalists' using such experience "until the news has played out." The Times also claims ownership to anything that appears in its publications or productions (New York Times Company 2005, 14).

New York Times staffers who host their own personal web pages or blogs are counseled that they cannot completely separate themselves from their professional connection with the Times. They are told that they "must avoid taking stands on divisive public issues." However separate the journalist believes the blog or website to be, the writing "must nevertheless be temperate in tone, reflecting taste, decency and respect for the dignity and privacy of others" (New York Times Company 2005, 13). In a world in which journalists have varied opportunities to contribute to the public discussion, news organizations have an affirmative duty to publish clear guidelines for employees that are also available to audience members.

Developing a sexual, romantic, or otherwise intimate relationship with a source is also considered to be a conflict of interest. While there may not be a financial component, sustaining a relationship that is in one's self-interest may take precedence over following one's news judgment. Similarly, the desire to produce an award-winning story or picture may interfere with news judgment. But, while news organizations can disallow close relationships with sources or require disclosure of relationships with potential newsmakers, it is more difficult to control an individual's drive for reward. But through initial training and appropriate prioritizing of values in the newsroom, journalists learn and are reminded that the goal is to produce great news, with the understanding that great news may be rewarded, rather than simply to produce the kind of stories that they hope will be rewarded. This kind of conflict is often more of an issue for visual journalists. Something that everyone in the newsroom agrees is "a helluva picture" may be published for its aesthetic or sensational value rather than for its newsworthiness.

It is not possible to entirely avoid conflicts of interest, nor does self-interest always conflict with professional interest. Most journalists strive to meet their role-related responsibilities and to do so without causing anyone unjustifiable harm. That is simply the ethical thing to do. However, most also appreciate the kudos and feeling of satisfaction that come from a job well done. Journalists need to get paid for the work they do. When professional interest and self-interest are complementary, the important individual responsibility is to put the professional interest first. Individual intentions in this regard are simply not accessible to others.

Conflicts of Interest for Institutions

News institutions can also be drawn into serving self-interest rather than the public interest. According to one study, "More than 40% of journalists and news executives surveyed admitted that they had engaged in self-censorship by purposely avoiding newsworthy stories or softening the tone of stories. With media organizations trying to attract more readers and larger audiences, market pressures were most often cited as the reason for such self-censorship . . . More than a third of all respondents said news that might hurt the financial interests of a news organization is sometimes or often ignored. More than one-third said they censored themselves because of personal career concerns" (Croteau and Hoynes 2005, 172).

News organizations have always had to make money. Even not-for-profit news entities could not stay in business without bringing in enough income to pay reporters and otherwise support news production. But the late twentieth century saw a shift from family ownership to corporate ownership and from news organizations owned by an entity that produced only news to ownership by conglomerates with a variety of interests. With corporate and conglomerate values came news managers who were hired precisely because they shared those values. "By the 1980's, the consolidation of media ownership put businesspeople, rather than journalists, in ultimate charge of news divisions" (Croteau and Hoynes 2005, 160).

Market pressures are discussed in the journalism ethics literature but are rarely labeled as the conflicts of interest that they are. For example, a story on the front page of the *New York Times* Arts section of December 4, 2007, says that "morning programs like 'Today' on NBC and 'The View' on ABC are the modern equivalents of the old Barbizon Hotel for Women, a frilly haven where men were not allowed above the first floor—or here, after the first hour—and viewers are treated to diet tips, ambush makeovers, cancer health scares, relationship counseling and, of course, shopping." These shows "have blurred the distinction between consumer news and product promotion." Despite a note that "it used to be that hosts who are part of the network's news division maintained an air of neutrality during consumer segments; now they are in on the pitch," the blurring is treated as an extension of the status quo: "Product placement is hardly a new phenomenon, and the morning shows long ago mastered the quid pro quo of daily television: Actors give interviews timed to their latest projects; authors are recruited as experts just as their books hit the stores" (Stanley 2007).

The tendency of media observers, along with owners and managers of news organizations, is simply to make note of how economic values are replacing news values. These observations are described but rarely judged in a normative way. To call these organizational conflicts of interest by name would imply that the organizations have an obligation to address the ethical implications of failing to meet their responsibilities to citizens. However, the conflict is clear. "The responsibility of journalism to report fully and fairly on events of the day has the potential to clash with the interests of corporate parents to promote their businesses and minimize any negative news about their operations. In addition, because their business interests are so broad and far-reaching, there are very few economic or legislative initiatives that do not affect some part of a media conglomerate" (Croteau and Hoynes 2005, 177).

In the light of journalism's commitment to timely truth-telling, news agents are ethically required to address interests and situations in which there is even an appearance of a conflict. The credibility of news media rests on citizens' assumptions that their favorite news source is choosing material based on no value deemed higher than the public interest and is presenting information in news contexts that is balanced, accurate, relevant, and complete (the BARC formula of news presentation). "Society is vulnerable to the judgment of journalists . . . we are highly dependent on journalists for furnishing information that enables us to make meaningful decisions about our lives, and we have little choice but to trust that journalists will strive to meet our needs and interests in this regard" (Borden and Pritchard 2001, 75). Anything that challenges this assumption weakens the credibility that separates journalism from other sources of information. But individual journalists are dependent on their news organization to provide the conflict-free latitude for them to do their own best work.

Just as individuals have conflicts of interest, news organizations have a combination of interests in making news and making money. Whether those interests are complementary or competing depends on leadership within the news organization. A classic example of an institutional conflict of interest is the case of the Los Angeles Times and Staples Center. In October 1999, the Los Angeles Times devoted a complete Sunday magazine issue to coverage of the newly opened Staples Center Arena. The journalists who worked on the issue did not know that news and business managers had secretly entered into an agreement with Staples Center owners to split the advertising profits from the magazine. Readers and reporters were appalled when this came to light, and top managers lost their jobs. But this was no accidental slip-up or surprising error in judgment. Instead, it was the culmination of the two-year reign of publisher Mark Willes, who "announced that he was dismantling the wall between the paper's business and editorial departments, saying he'd blow it up with a 'bazooka' if necessary. Willes contended that the two could work together to help the paper, without allowing advertisers to influence news decisions" (Croteau and Hoynes 2005, 164).

As egregious as it was for the Los Angeles Times to be so closely entwined with a potential news source, some forms of "ad-formation" are common-place. For example, most newspapers have "special" sections. According to Croteau and Hoynes (2006, 168), "At the Oregonian, the advertiser-friendly home and auto sections are simply written by the ad department. The Denver Post turns over the production of its skiing, gardening, casino gambling, and other sections to its advertising department." In the absence of convention, rule, or disclosure, few readers know whether the food section is sponsored by advertisers or is produced by reporters in the newsroom. It is not unusual for local weather pieces on local news programs to have local sponsors. No one outside the newsroom knows whether the piece on the local hospital's latest diagnostic tool was really produced as news or the television station is running a video news release produced by the hospital's public relations department in the hope of generating business for the new and expensive machine. The lack of transparency by news organizations in this regard can create a suspicion of a conflict of interest. Audience members simply do not know whether the institution is putting their or the sponsor's interests first. As even the appearance of a conflict erodes journalistic credibility, news organizations have an obligation to separate advertising and sponsorship from all news production. It is ethically required that they explicitly tell audience members when advertising interests and news production are combined.

Conflicts of interest can develop simply because it is cheaper for news organizations to accept what they are given by sources in the form of press releases, video news releases, and photo opportunities, rather than to have journalists conduct independent and time-consuming investigations. Ac-

cording to Croteau and Haynes (2005, 163), "Commercial news organizations would like to produce credible news coverage at the lowest possible cost.
This leads to practices in which journalists rely on outside sources to feed
them stories. Routine news material from government and the private sector
efficiently helps news organizations fill their broadcasts and newspapers." As
the least powerful elements of the community have the least access to marketing techniques and knowledge, they are the least likely to be represented in
the pursuit of cheap news production. When news organizations ignore the
need of the powerless to have a voice, the whole community suffers. Citizens
do not get all the information they need to have for self-governance when the
voice of the least powerful is ignored.

Another development that creates potential conflicts is that of "transaction journalism," in which journalistic accounts are tied to the promotion of
products. "For example, next to its book reviews, the online edition of the
New York Times . . . carries a direct link to an online bookseller, in this case
barnesandnoble.com . . . The New York Times gets a percentage of the book's
sale price for having brought the consumer to the barnesandnoble.com site.
Because a negative review is unlikely to generate sales, the newspaper now
has a financial interest in promoting—rather than just reviewing—a book"
(Croteau and Hoynes 2005, 169).

And, while the combining of journalism with advertising interests might
be an obvious trap for institutions to avoid, there is also the more subtle trend
toward making news more entertaining to boost numbers of readers or viewers
and therefore increase sales. "Sex, violence, spectacle: these sorts of programs
are the logical end products of the corporate pursuit of profits. They are relatively cheap to produce and, like an accident on the highway, they predictably
draw a regular audience. What these programs lack, however, is any sense of
serving a larger public interest by providing substantive content" (Croteau and
Hoynes 2005, 157). In the conventional vernacular of local television news,
"If it bleeds, it leads." The most visually dramatic story is far more likely to be
the featured news package at the top of a program than the story that is more
relevant to self-governance and, predictably, less dramatic.

Advertising, entertainment values, and news all come together when the
focus of news managers is pleasing the audience or serving up what audience
members say they want, rather than providing what is most in the public interest. "The result can be feel-good, watered-down sensationalized news that
may attract readers and audiences, but that leaves citizens with little of substance. Citizens wind up with 'news' that serves commercial interests rather

than the public interest. Managers are rewarded for increased profitability while journalists are left wondering what has happened to their 'profession'" (Croteau and Hoynes 2005, 164).

Institutions have a responsibility to refrain from conflicts of interest or the appearance of conflicts of interest. When it is not possible to refrain—such as the need for a news organization to make a profit in addition to fulfilling its ethical responsibility—for the sake of credibility, the news organization needs to be transparent with its audience about how it is handling the conflict. It is not enough to note the drift in the industry from news values to commercial values. Just as for-profit hospitals have a responsibility to provide high-quality patient care despite the interests of the stockholders, so do news organizations have a responsibility to provide information that citizens need for self-governance, regardless of economic interest.

Conflicts of Commitment for Individuals and Institutions

Even the most self-aware individuals and institutions will have conflicts of commitment. Individual journalists' conflicts of commitment most often arise in the social activism arena. It is natural that journalists should be passionate about political issues and social justice. *Caring* about the news is certainly an essential element to gathering and reporting the news. However, many news organizations and individual journalists have a hard time determining where to draw the line in civic participation. Marching in a pro-choice or pro-life rally is generally not allowed; contributing to a cause, particularly if the contribution is anonymous, often is allowed. Having campaign signs in one's front yard is generally not allowed; voting is permitted.

The closer one's personal connection to a newsworthy matter, the more difficult it becomes to justify covering the story. For example, a city hall reporter and a photographer for the San Francisco Chronicle were taken off coverage of "marriage for gays and lesbians, because they were among the thousands of same-sex couples who received marriage licenses through the city." The determination was made on the basis "that *Chronicle* journalists directly and personally involved in a major news story—one in whose outcome they also have a personal stake—should not also cover that story" (McBride 2008, 1–2).

Personal involvement in a story damages the journalist's ability to be unbiased or to be perceived by the audience as unbiased. But so does public political and civic involvement. The question is not *whether* journalists are allowed to participate in matters of social importance. It is, rather, whether journalists should be allowed *additional* participation in matters of social importance. Journalists are active in the community by nature of doing their jobs. Additional participation gives them additional power above that which they already enjoy; and as the power of the personal rides on the coattails of the news organization, it is impossible to effectively separate the two.

Journalists should give up the opportunity for additional political and civic involvement for the sake of their own and their news organization's credibility. Journalists are not the only professionals who need to restrict their off-hours' activities because of how those activities might reflect on their employers or on public perception of their work. Imagine a judge demonstrating against the death penalty, or an employee of the Environmental Protection Agency arguing against clean air and water standards.

Institutional conflicts of commitment arise when the role of the news organization as good corporate citizen is considered. News organizations, for example, are often involved in local philanthropy, from having their own "People in Need" or "Send a Kid to Camp" funds and accompanying stories to involvement in the local United Way campaign. While it is not wrong for corporations to support their local communities, news organizations that do so can run the risk of interfering with their journalists' ability to conduct independent reporting. Nothing in the community should be above scrutiny. Nonprofit status, or approval as a United Way agency, does not imply that a charity is "good." Social service agencies can fail to meet the needs of their clients. Philanthropic organizations can be the site of scandal and misuse of funds. But careful journalistic scrutiny of a cultural or philanthropic or social service organization is less likely to happen if the news organization's owner, publisher, or station manager serves on its board.

Most troublesome in this regard is the role that United Way plays in most newsrooms. "Of all the charities and non-profits that exist within a community, only United Way gets the benefit of widespread payroll deductions. Few fund drives involve reporters receiving pledge cards with their paychecks. Even fewer can boast of newsroom 'volunteers' who follow up with colleagues, checking to ensure that everyone has 'had the opportunity to give'" (Elliott 1991). United Way implicitly gets managerial approval that results in newspapers and programs that keep track of the success of the fund-raising drives, with plenty of stories to encourage citizens to give. United Way, and the agencies under its wing, receives little journalistic scrutiny. Just as it is reasonable to expect journalists to refrain from involvement in political and civic activity that would call the credibility of the news organization into question, I believe it is reasonable to expect news organizations, and their managers, to refrain from involvement with outside organizations that then come to be viewed in the newsroom as exempt from scrutiny.

Attachment to government can also be a problem. It is conventionally understood that journalism serves as the "watchdog" on government. Part of what citizens need to know for self-governance is what government is doing in our name and any controversies regarding those actions. Participating in the military's "embedded journalism" program may be the only way to cover war in real time. But when news anchors wear American-flag lapel pins and newspapers print full-color, full-page flags to display in one's window, news organizations are failing to meet the public interest. In a time of national crisis, citizens need news organizations that critically report our government's actions and how they are being perceived in a global context. Citizens do not need journalism that simply repeats government officials' perspectives or that panders to the latest public opinion poll.

Equally troublesome, but conventionally accepted, is the role of news organizations in endorsing candidates or voter initiatives or weighing in on controversial civic matters through editorials. Along with offering a public forum for citizens' and external commentators' opinions, news organizations present their own well-reasoned arguments in favor of or against a variety of public issues. While most news organizations erect a "wall" between those who write for the news side and those who write editorials, the separation is not apparent to audience members. It is not unreasonable for audience members to wonder about the ability of a journalist to remain unbiased when, seemingly, the news organization as a whole is throwing its weight on one side or another of a campaign or controversy.

Conclusion

Traditionally, news organizations have dealt swiftly with individual reporters who violated conflict-of-interest policies. Reporters were either fired or reassigned to eliminate even the appearance that journalists might have covered stories with which they had a strong connection. Elimination of journalistic bias has traditionally been viewed as essential to the news organization's maintaining its credibility.

As strict as news organizations have generally been, however, in dealing with individual reporters' conflicts of interest, the organizations have been equally lax regarding potential conflicts at the executive or organizational level. This expression of selective attention has created a perception of mixed messages, at best, and an unwillingness to address the systematic conflicts of interest.

As with other professions and societal practices, news organizations are fraught with potentially conflicting situations. Many people, passions, and principles can pull at individuals and institutions that are working to serve the public interest. The advantage that news organizations have, but rarely use, is the ability to communicate directly and easily with those they serve. Disclosure of competing interests ought to come early and often, along with management's explanation of how potential conflicts, particularly at the institutional level, are being handled.

REFERENCES

Borden, S. L., and M. S. Pritchard. 2001. Conflict of interest in journalism. In *Conflict of Interest in the Professions*, ed. M. Davis and A. Stark, 73–91. New York: Oxford University Press.

Bugeja, M. 2008. *Living Ethics across Media Platforms*. New York: Oxford University Press

Croteau, D., and W. Hoynes. 2005. *The Business of Media, Corporate Media, and the Public Interest*. Thousand Oaks, CA: Pine Forge Press.

Dicken-Garcia, H. 1989. *Journalistic Standards in Nineteenth-Century America*. Madison: University of Wisconsin Press.

Elliott, D. 1991. How now, sacred cow? United Way's favored treatment by media. *FineLine: The Newsletter on Journalism Ethics* 3 (1): 4.

Englehardt, E. E., and R. D. Barney. 1999. *Media and Ethics: Principles for Moral Decisions*. New York: Wadsworth.

Kovach, B., and T. Rosenstiel. 2007. *The Elements of Journalism (Revised)*. New York: Three Rivers Press.

McBride, K. 2008. Searching for the threshold. *Poynter Ethics Journal*, June 16. www.poynter.org.

National Press Photographers Association. 2006. *NPPA Code of Ethics*. Durham, NC: National Press Photographers Association. www.nppa.org.

New York Times Company. 2005. *The New York Times Company Policy on Ethics in Journalism*. New York: New York Times Company. www.nytco.com/press/ethics.html.

Radio-Television News Directors Association and Foundation. 2000. *Code of Ethics and Professional Conduct, Radio-Television News Directors Assocation*. Washington, DC: Radio-Television News Directors Association and Foundation. www.rtnda.org.

Society of Professional Journalists. 1996. *Society of Professional Journalists Code of Ethics*. Indianapolis, IN: Society of Professional Journalists. www.spj.org/ethicscode.asp.

Stanley, A. 2007. Morning TV veers from news to frills. *New York Times*, Dec. 4.

Werhane and Doering. 1996. Conflicts of interest and conflicts of commitment. *Professional Ethics, a Multidisciplinary Journal* 4 (3&4): 47–81.

CHAPTER 8

Some Principles Require Principals

Why Banning "Conflicts of Interest" Won't Solve Incentive Problems in Biomedical Research

WILLIAM M. SAGE, M.D., J.D.

Money seems to have supplanted state power as the principal concern of biomedical research ethics. Each year brings new illustrations of the tension between financial flows and the moral and legal duties of academic biomedical researchers.

- A young man dies after university-based physicians with a commercial stake in a novel gene therapy ignore warning signs when enrolling research participants to test the procedure (Stolberg 1999).
- A pharmaceutical company pressures a university to which it has promised a large gift to demote a researcher who published research casting the company's products in a negative light (Rennie 1997).
- A pharmaceutical company attempts to prevent a university researcher from reporting that, contrary to expectations, its proprietary formulation of a human hormone is not superior to cheaper generics (Rennie 1997; *In re Synthroid Marketing Litigation*, 264 F.3d 712, 714 [7th Cir. 2001]).
- Another pharmaceutical company pressures university researchers with whom it has contracts not to publish findings that antidepressant drugs are ineffective and may increase the risk of suicide (Meier 2004).
- A prominent health care provider conducts clinical trials on a new use of a Food and Drug Administration (FDA)–approved radiofrequency ablation device in which the health care provider itself and its physician-CEO have invested, publishes its results in peer-reviewed journals,

and treats more than a thousand patients with the device "off-label" (Armstrong 2005).

Criticism of financial relationships of this sort has been widespread, with individuals, organizations, associations, and government entities universally labeling them "conflicts of interest." This chapter challenges the legal and ethical language of such an accusation and the implications of that language—not the underlying need for current action or future vigilance. As it is typically employed in biomedical ethical commentary, the term *conflict of interest* mixes specific obligations to identifiable patients with general ideals of conduct that are vulnerable to a host of human frailties (Krimsky 2003, 27–56).

I argue here that a conflict-of-interest framework is inappropriate for protecting the abstract integrity of biomedical research, which would be better achieved through direct regulation of financial incentives. On the other hand, conflict-of-interest analysis may help define the obligations of biomedical researchers (and clinicians) to their academic employers. Making individual behavior consistent with institutional mission also may shed light on the multiple roles played by academic health systems in patient care, research, and teaching, reveal tensions among them, and promote more responsible conduct with respect to patients, sponsors, and communities.

Incoherent "Conflict-of-Interest" Discourse in Biomedical Research

A distinction needs to be made between two different kinds of obligation: one involving identifiable persons (patients, research participants, employers) to whom loyalty is owed, the other implicating primarily general concepts of principled science and medicine. As the term is used by lawyers describing their own professional responsibilities, a conflict of interest is a fiduciary construct that has clear meaning only within a relational framework, meaning one person's responsibility for another. From this perspective, one can define the term as follows: "A conflict of interest arises when a person (the agent) stands in a relationship of trust with another person (the principal) that requires the agent to exercise judgment on behalf of the principal, and where the agent's judgment is impaired because of another interest of the agent" (Wendel 2003, 477). This approach is suited to legal and ethical oversight of conflicts of interest involving professionals who owe duties to identifiable clients or other individuals. Accordingly, most entanglements that trouble scholars of conflicts of interest in the professional context are those that potentially compromise judgment and conduct in discrete relationships or transactions.

In contrast to the legal scholar's relational definition of conflicts of interest, medical commentators posit a broader range of problematic behaviors. Consider Denis Thompson's definition of conflict of interest (1993, 573), which is the starting point for most bioethical commentary: "a set of conditions in which professional judgment concerning a primary interest (such as a patient's welfare or the validity of research) tends to be unduly influenced by a secondary interest (such as financial gain)." Following this approach, most discussions fail to specify a principal party to whom the researcher's fidelity is owed and do not distinguish relational obligations from generally desirable behavior among researchers. Yet the remedies that these same commentators recommend, such as disclosure and segregation of functions, are based on an unacknowledged relational paradigm.

Thompson's example of a patient's welfare is a relational obligation for that patient's treating physician. His other example, the validity of research, is not relational, at least vis-à-vis the patient. Conducting valid research may well be a relational obligation for a researcher who is employed by a university or pharmaceutical company, but it runs only to the employer, not to research study participants. Using the same term—conflict of interest—to foster both an employee's loyalty to an employer and the employee's social consciousness is misleading. Suppression by a company researcher of internally generated findings, release of which would reduce the company's profitability, honors her obligation to her employer, yet may be contrary to the public interest. This is not a "conflict of interest" but something else—perhaps a violation of an independent legal obligation placed on the company to make results public or a lack of personal ethical commitment to "do the right thing" on the researcher's part.

Distinguishing Relational and Regulatory Obligations in Bioethics

An irony of current biomedical research regulation is that its founding documents were largely a moral reaction to government abuses: the Nuremberg Code, a response to human experimentation by Nazi Germany, and the Belmont Report, a response to the U.S. Public Health Service's Tuskegee syphilis study. Government, however, now plays the central role in protecting human subjects from the research professionals whom it funds. Correspond-ingly, ethicists have shifted their concern from policing government to ensur-ing that scientists fulfill both relational obligations to research participants and nonrelational social responsibilities to the public that supports them.

Conflict-of-interest analysis in biomedical research typically operates un-der the presumption that the principal party to whom loyalty is owed is the patient or research participant (DuVal 2004). Conflict-of-interest analysis makes sense in an ethics regime that focuses on individual researchers' (espe-cially clinician-researchers') professionalism when balancing research goals with patient care goals. Informed consent, for example, was described by early bioethicists as a personal, relational task.

By contrast, modern research ethics is alert to the danger of therapeutic misconception and seeks to disabuse research participants of the notion that researchers are primarily concerned with participants' personal medical outcomes. A system that focuses on the social benefits and costs of biomedi-cal research—even if highly protective of research participants' safety and autonomy—is principle-based, rather than principal-based. A principle-based approach to research ethics and governance reduces the coherence of conflict-of-interest discourse and renders traditional devices for ensuring personal loyalty, such as disclosure or prohibition, less compatible with socially desir-able outcomes.

Dignitary obligations of researchers to research participants, such as re-specting personhood and protecting physical safety, remain important even in a principled rather than "principaled" system. Enforcing these duties, how-ever, does not require the strict fiduciary analysis that is necessary to make conflicts of interest meaningful. There are also direct relational obligations from physicians to their patients in many clinical research settings. "Conflict of interest" retains meaning under these conditions, but it cannot alone de-termine the professional responsibilities of the physician-researcher.

Recognizing that complex public-private arrangements, not personal rela-tionships between research physicians and patient-subjects, increasingly de-fine the modern biomedical research enterprise also brings needed scrutiny to the roles and responsibilities of contemporary academic institutions. Several important questions arise. First, what relational obligations do these institu-tions owe to other parties (e.g., patients, sponsors, communities) as agents or fiduciaries? Second, how are competing obligations to be fulfilled or recon-ciled? Third, what overarching regulatory responsibilities does academic bio-medicine have to the public? Finally, can clarifying the relational duties owed by individuals working in biomedical research settings to their institutional employers—a pragmatic trend that seems to be emerging—help provide overall assurances of productive, ethical research?

Confusing Conflicts of Interest with Incentives

A source of confusion in the biomedical research context is the tendency to equate incentives with conflicts of interest. Conflict-of-interest terminology is ill equipped to divide acceptable from unacceptable motives and motivators in the absence of specific relational obligations. Commentators such as Norman Levinsky (2002) correctly point out that a medical researcher, or anyone else for that matter, can be driven to achieve by the prospect of advancement, peer approval, public acclaim, family esteem, and many other things, in addition to cash.

The difficulty is that these vague motives can just as easily align as misalign the incentives of researchers with those of parties whose relational interests they arguably might serve—whether patients, institutional employers, or funders. That these incentives exist is generally a good thing, no matter to what principal party a researcher is thought to owe primary responsibility. The alternative, particularly for academics with tenure, is a generation of complacent, self-absorbed, unproductive scientists. For this reason, among others, unfocused science has largely given way to targeted support, regardless of whether the research sponsor is a commercial, private nonprofit, or government entity (Belsky and Emanuel 2004, 268, 270).

Incentives matter, and they are challenging to get right in any principal-agent relationship. Why do critics of academic-industry relationships not recognize this? One detectable undercurrent in the critical literature is moral judgment. Commentators seem to be looking for "pure-hearted" professionals—researchers whose *raison d'être* is to pursue the ideals of science (Krimsky 2003, 230). One practical consequence of this preference is to draw bright lines between corruptible and incorruptible scientists, rather than assessing the degree of risk to judgment posed by specific arrangements. Another is to regard all commercial involvement by suspect sources as temptation to evil. Blanket prohibitions on contact between pharmaceutical companies and physicians, for example, fail to distinguish between interns who eat pizza paid for by drug detailers and department chairs who accept tens of thousands of dollars in cash.

A parallel problem is that real life seldom conforms to the expectations of moralists. No biomedical researcher is an island. Critics of conflicts of interest acknowledge that financial relationships are widespread in medicine and therefore cannot all be bad, but they still freely condemn particular examples (Barnes and Florencio 2002). This has the effect of favoring the familiar for little reason beyond its familiarity. Medical journals, for example, were quick to criticize university scientists for accepting industry subsidies that could bias research and immediately imposed financial disclosure obligations on their contributing authors. However, those journals have no qualms about their established practice of publishing articles without payment to the authors, making it inevitable that support for those articles will be provided by the authors' employers or third parties.

Mapping Relational Duties in Biomedical Research

How might one perform a systematic analysis of conflicts of interest in biomedical research? One way to recognize inconsistencies in current policy is to identify potential principals and agents in the research environment. If one can do so, then one can assert primary obligations of loyalty against which conflicts of interest can be measured. If one cannot do so, then it is a pretty good bet that, even if real tensions and risks exist in biomedical research, conflict-of-interest analysis is the wrong conceptual tool with which to solve those problems.

By way of comparison, lawyers' ethics takes a disciplined approach to identifying and classifying conflicts of interest involving the "client" (the principal to whom the lawyer owes undivided allegiance as agent), the lawyer, and others—including third parties who might be paying for the lawyer's services. If one analyzes conflicts of interest in research as a lawyer would, only three basic professional-client-payer permutations are available to map the research landscape surrounding an individual biomedical scientist: research participant as client, university employer as client, and research sponsor as client. The first two possibilities are discussed below and are explored in detail elsewhere (Sage 2007b). The first fails to anchor a successful governing structure for conflicts of interest in biomedical research. The second provides a workable template for day-to-day institutional policies but suffers from major conceptual gaps and operational ambiguities. The third either reinforces the need for regulation to constrain private duty (in cases of commercial sponsorship or research) or essentially duplicates a regulatory regime (in cases of government sponsorship).

Lawyers' Relational Ethics and Conflicts of Interest

The approach to conflicts of interest taken in the regulation and self-regulation of lawyers can serve a clarifying function for biomedical research. In the typical account of legal ethics, "role morality" for lawyers means the primacy of the single client's interest (Haskell 1998, 35–38). This duty of loyalty includes, as core values, "zealous" advocacy, confidentiality regarding both facts and communications, and nonexploitation (American Bar Association 2007).

Legal ethics addresses three types of conflict of interest that threaten such loyalty. The first category encompasses "client-client" conflicts, involving competing positions and interests between current or former clients of the lawyer. These are the most commonly discussed and the most routinely prevented or addressed conflicts of interest in law, but in other fields they are sometimes described as "conflicts of commitment" (Epstein 1992; Werhane and Doering 1997, 165). The second category encompasses "client-lawyer" conflicts involving lawyer self-dealing or misappropriation. The third category encompasses "client-payer" conflicts, in which someone other than the client (e.g., the client's liability insurer) pays for services to the client and seeks to control those services. Within modern law firms employing many lawyers, client-client conflicts that would disqualify one lawyer are imputed to the firm as a whole in most instances, but client-lawyer conflicts generally are limited to situations in which the lawyer with the conflict is personally serving the client.

It is noteworthy that legal ethics does not automatically condemn conflicts of interest unless they are unidentified and therefore unmanaged. Rather, conflicts are understood to be omnipresent risks of legal professionalism. Depending on the type of conflict, management can take several forms. One common approach is client consent after disclosure and, sometimes, required consultation with independent counsel. This is typical for client-lawyer conflicts and often includes a substantive review for fairness. Outright prohibition occurs in some client-client conflicts, typically involving opposing parties in ongoing litigation. A third approach, common within law firms but rarely endorsed by ethical codes, attempts to isolate lawyers serving one group of clients from other lawyers serving clients with conflicting interests.

Law has also developed a range of remedies for conflicts violations. One straightforward, effective remedy that compensates a disadvantaged client while also punishing and deterring misconduct is disgorgement of legal fees collected during representations that fail to comply with rules of professional responsibility. In more serious cases, counsel can be disqualified during representation. Because conflicts rules are explicit and essential components of mandatory professional codes for lawyers, formal disciplinary action up to and including disbarment is possible, a remedy that emphasizes protecting future clients rather than aiding current clients. Legal malpractice suits seeking monetary damages may be available also, but these require proof that the violation of the conflicts rule caused measurable harm to the plaintiff.

To facilitate comparison with biomedicine, it is also important to appreciate that substantial tensions in client representation are not addressed by lawyers' formal conflict-of-interest rules. First, conflicts between lawyers' service to their clients and lawyers' personal beliefs and moral commitments are discussed in the codes of professional responsibility but resist clear rules beyond a permissive approach to withdrawing from representation. Second, lawyers' public duties are not considered part of conflict-of-interest analysis. Lawyers, particularly in litigation, are charged as "officers of the court" and have enforceable, though limited, responsibilities not to subvert the adversary system. Significantly, only narrow obligations associated with specific situations are part of the mandatory rules of professional conduct. General obligations such as to serve "justice," however laudable, are expressed in hortatory terms, if at all (American Bar Association 2007).

A final point essential to understanding the appropriate scope of biomedical conflicts of interest is that the *incentives* that induce a lawyer to undertake a particular representation are almost always distinct from conflicts of interest. Incentives include practices such as accepting cases for litigation on contingency, with attorney fees payable as a percentage of a successful recovery, and taking equity stakes in transactional clients in lieu of hourly fees or cash retainers. No financial arrangements between lawyers and clients—or, for that matter, between any principal and any agent—perfectly align incentives. Each attorney fee structure mixes effective with perverse incentives and must be evaluated and refined periodically. Fee arrangements are discussed, and occasionally restricted, in lawyers' rules of professional conduct. Beyond cross-references, however, their regulation is separate from the regulation of conflicts of interest.

Why Research Participants Are Not "Clients" in Biomedical Research

One plausible permutation of agency relationships in biomedical research is to position the research participant as the researcher's "client." Translating from research terms into lawyers' terms, the public or private research sponsor would be cast as the payer for services to the client, other participants and patients would be either joint or competing clients, and the academic health center would be analogous to a law firm.

The logical problem with considering the research participant the principal party in a supposed principal-agent relationship is that, in biomedical research, the putative beneficiary, by definition, would not be able to benefit from the activity. Recent conceptions of research ethics hold that the only benefit that accrues to a research participant is altruistic gain from contributing to a socially useful enterprise (Appelbaum 2002). Labeling the research participant a "principal party" creates a paradox. Equating the participant's physical well-being with his or her interests leads to the conclusion that any goal of research contrary to the interests of the participant in avoiding physical harm is a conflict of interest, which is clearly unworkable. Equating the participant's altruism with his or her interests leads to the equally illogical conclusion that no conflict of interest arises if the research furthers "sound science." This is not to say that researchers owe no duties to participants, just that participants cannot logically occupy the role of principal in the sort of agency relationship that is amenable to conflicts analysis.

If individual "representation" of research participants by researchers is impractical, might researchers represent participants in the aggregate? Legal ethics generally disfavors group representation. Although class-action and mass-tort lawyers represent groups of plaintiffs in litigation, and although group representation by medical professionals is possible, research participants cannot form a "corporate client" and do not naturally share interests. Even in a specific study, individuals may participate for different reasons and hold different preferences regarding risks and procedures. Ultimately, the idea of representing research participants as a group converges with serving the public interest in sound but safe science, which, as I argue in this chapter, is not amenable to governance in relational terms.

Institutions as Research "Clients"

In the abstract, other principal-agent combinations could be structured into the legal governance of biomedical research. One option conceives of the academic center as the client of individual researchers and therefore the party to whom they are loyal and by whom they are paid. Considering the ubiquity of employment relationships in biomedical research, academic health centers and other nonprofit health care organizations might construct conflict-of-interest policies to ensure that clinicians and researchers in their employ remain loyal to them.

A trend toward academic health centers policing the conduct of individual researchers and clinicians seems to be emerging. In 2008, for example, a task force of the Association of American Medical Colleges (AAMC) issued a detailed report to the organization's executive council suggesting that member organizations place strict controls on their physician-employees' contact with the pharmaceutical and medical device industries (Association of American Medical Colleges 2008). Although the report, perhaps intentionally, refrains from describing the proscribed behavior as disloyalty to the institutional employer, the effect of the task force's recommendations is to replicate an approach to conflict of interest as familiar to corporate America as it seems unfamiliar to academic medicine—a fact driven home to me by an exchange at the Hastings Center conference that launched this book. Following two days of animated conversation, mainly focused on the need to reduce the financial influence of the pharmaceutical industry on biomedicine, the conference host thanked the participants and reminded them to send him their travel expenses to be reimbursed from grant funds provided by a charitable foundation. One, and only one, participant immediately declined reimbursement: the director of ethics and compliance for a major pharmaceutical company. An employee accepting travel funds from a third party, she explained, would violate her company's conflict-of-interest policy.

Nonetheless, reconstructing biomedical institutional relationships in this fashion may run into practical difficulties. One constraint is that research universities typically have decentralized governance, which both derives from and reinforces notions of academic freedom. Another problem is the mixed missions of biomedical institutions, including research, education, and clinical care (Korn 1996). This amalgam of objectives is problematic from a relational perspective. Using the same clinical infrastructure for research, teaching, and clinical care may subject the academic setting to irreconcilable conflicts similar to those raised in the recent debate over lawyers' participation in "multidisciplinary practices" that would share duties and governance among professions and nonprofessional disciplines with varying responsibilities and ethical priorities.

Institutional conflicts of interest have received scant attention until relatively recently. According to an AAMC task force report, "an institution may have a conflict of interest in human subjects research whenever the financial interests of the institution, or of an institutional official acting within his or her authority . . . might affect—or reasonably appear to affect—institutional processes for the conduct, review, or oversight of human subjects research" (AAMC Task Force on Financial Conflicts of Interest in Clinical Research 2002, 2). Like many statements on the topic, this commentary subsumes within "conflict of interest" several institutional roles and does not distinguish among them. An academic health center has various compliance obligations, both to government directly and to self-regulatory organizations, but it is not particularly helpful to describe them as vulnerable to conflicts of interest. On the other hand, academic health centers routinely perform functions to which law attaches specific relational duties, such as caring for patients, and assume other relational obligations by voluntary agreement, such as accepting research grants. One set of such activities may indeed constitute a conflict of interest with another set, and all may be vulnerable to conflicts with other institutional interests, such as the financial concerns of the general university that often controls an academic health center.

An additional obstacle to demanding that researchers be loyal to their university employers is that nonprofit enterprises seldom pay full freight to their faculty from institutional funds as salaries and benefits. As a result, they tolerate and even endorse the pursuit of outside remuneration that has the effect of supporting the academic mission. At the University of Texas at Austin (2007), for example, general staff members are cautioned not to accept payments from external sources, but the university's official policy for faculty states that "faculty are *encouraged* to seek remunerative outside employment" that does not compromise their teaching duties or use university resources. A conflict-of-interest policy emphasizing institutional loyalty is incompatible with this pattern of cross-subsidies.

These tensions are beginning to surface in both consensus statements and individual institutional policies but have not yet been resolved or even fully acknowledged. For example, institutional conflict-of-interest policies often start by addressing the personal interests of "institutional officials" who have the power to bind the university (AAMC Task Force on Financial Conflicts of Interest in Clinical Research 2002). Misappropriation by insiders is a real risk in all organizations, but universities have less centralized decision-making than most other corporate entities, and the deeper problem is the conflict inherent in the institution's own interests. Solutions thus far have emphasized "firewalls" between financial and scientific decisions, which would be considered an inadequate remedy in any other corporate context. A dramatic example, from clinical medicine rather than research, is the clear recognition that individual physicians should not both treat potential organ donors and transplant donated organs into recipients, but lack of attention to the possibility that both sets of physicians are employed by the same organization.

Policing by universities of employed physicians or scientists is also becoming more common but remains tentative. Restrictions are usually justified on the supposedly altruistic (and often paternalistic) grounds of reducing risk of scientific bias rather than on the pragmatic, and more clearly defined, grounds of demanding loyalty to the institution (Association of American Medical Colleges 2008). So far, this has resulted in policies that risk being either too lax or too strict. An example of the former is the tendency to regard public disclosure as a cure-all, even when the institution's own duties to patients or third parties are not so easily waived. An example of the latter is the recommendation that universities prohibit employed physicians from attending sponsored pharmaceutical lectures outside working hours, which arguably is a First Amendment violation if enforced by a public entity.

Recasting "Conflicts" as Regulated Incentives

What does this analysis tell us? That there is no single principal party to whom biomedical researchers can demonstrate loyalty and therefore no logical foundation for constructing policies based on conflicts of interest. Research participants, however deserving of protection and respect, cannot occupy the principal's position. Employees' loyalty to employers may be a workable framework for individual institutions but remains insufficiently developed to anchor a general mechanism for legal and ethical governance. A more effective system of regulating for research incentives would shed the relational pretense.

One can respect research participants' personhood, rights, and interests without using principal-agent language. Modern research ethics takes a much more legalistic, regulatory approach than its relational, largely self-regulatory predecessor, a trend that an obsession with "conflict of interest" threatens to reverse. The basic goal of research regulation is to maximize the output of ethical research for a given level of funding. The Bayh-Dole Act of 1980, for example, was at root an exercise in off-budget, incentive-based regulation intended to facilitate technology transfer and therefore research productivity.

Placing public regulatory duties on biomedical researchers, including physicians, simply subjects their traditional role-governed ethics to additional rules of conduct. Physicians have always had public-interested as well as patient-interested duties. Recognizing this, medical ethics gives physicians greater freedom to limit relational duties to patients than is the case for lawyers and clients. Few parallels exist in clinical medicine to the client-client conflicts of interest that play a large role in lawyers' ethics; payers are allowed a more directive function in medicine than in law; and confidentiality rules are more often waived to allow physicians to benefit third parties or to further broad social objectives. Specialization in biomedical research makes a regulatory approach easier, because there is less likelihood of interfering with the relational obligations of the physician to his or her patient. Industrialization has similar effects: research institutions are an efficient focus for regulatory efforts, whereas it is hard to enforce detailed regulations against a large number of individual professionals.

Other expert economic sectors, including law and accounting, have also been forced to navigate a transition from self-governing profession to regulated industry. The Sarbanes-Oxley Act of 2002, for example, imposes regulatory duties on auditors (by banning corporate consulting income in order to further their obligation to report objectively to the public) and on lawyers (by relaxing strict standards of client confidentiality when financial fraud is at issue). Specialization and industrialization of these professions has facilitated regulation. Not every lawyer is a securities lawyer; not every accountant audits public companies. Those performing such functions, however, subject themselves to regulatory as well as relational monitoring. For those in regulated specialties such as law and accounting, moreover, the rules apply to law firms and accounting firms as institutions as well as to individual lawyers and auditors.

Calibrating Incentives for Productivity in Research

Shifting from conflict-of-interest discourse and other relational constructs to explicit public regulation of biomedical researchers has several potential benefits. Without the rhetorical distraction of parsing "conflicts of interest," public regulation can examine the complete picture of medical research and can calibrate incentives to stimulate desirable behavior. A public regulator can establish benchmarks for research quality and productivity and can assess empirically the extent of financial relationships involving biomedical researchers and the measurable harm arising from those relationships

(Steinbrook 2005). By contrast, there is no general "efficiency defense" to a conflict-of-interest violation cast in relational terms, because under traditional statements of fiduciary law and ethics, principal parties are entitled to categorically undivided loyalty.

A similar transition from relational to regulatory focus is already occurring with respect to the ethical analysis of payments to individuals serving as human subjects in biomedical research. Rather than condemning payment in relational terms as "undue influence," ethicists increasingly focus on the need to adequately incentivize participation in research—including by vulnerable populations that historically have had less access to medical innovations—and to rely instead on substantive regulation to ensure that the risks imposed on paid participants are reasonable in the light of the potential benefits to society of the research taking place (Emanuel 2004; Sage 2007a).

Building on baseline measurements, a regulator can model the effects on research outcomes of alternative policies that influence the balance of competitive and cooperative incentives affecting researchers and research institutions. How, for example, do direct cash payments from industry sponsors to individual researchers compare with deferred compensation through equity interests and patent royalties, focused grant support of research departments, and general support of academic institutions in terms of quantity of research produced, reliability of results, and ethical treatment of human subjects? If owner-innovators are permitted to test their inventions in human subjects at their own institutions, do the products turn out better or worse? Are the research participants safer or less safe? How much will it cost to partition research from treatment functions to prevent divided loyalties? Regulatory approaches, unlike many relational ones, allow empirics to matter.

Reputational Intermediaries and Self-Regulation

Even in a regulated environment, self-governance remains necessary and desirable to reinforce norms of proper conduct, adjust to changing conditions, and leverage public enforcement resources. Analyzing financial relationships in relational terms makes self-regulation susceptible to oversimplification of remedies and generational in-fighting. With incentives regulated through public processes directed at achieving explicit public objectives, self-regulation can work in more constructive ways.

Self-regulation is often invoked by critics of research commercialization.

Brennan and colleagues (2006), for example, call for "more stringent regulation" but envision most restrictions being imposed through self-regulatory processes rather than through direct government intervention. They propose a leadership role for academic medical centers, though they do not clearly distinguish among contract-based relational claims that such institutions have on the physicians and researchers they employ, contractual and fiduciary relational claims that patients have on academic medical centers, and the institutions' legal and ethical obligations to the public at large. Similarly, Greg Koski (2003), former director of the Office of Human Research Protections, believes that self-regulation, backed by the threat of severe government sanctions in "the most egregious cases," will increase acceptance of the underlying principles and focus scientists on preventing ethical lapses.

One possibility is the deliberate use of reputational intermediaries in the biomedical research environment (Coffee 2004). Organizations that endorse research results for public use are well positioned to monitor incentive structures and ensure that individual research scientists are responding in the desired ways. Universities and scientific journals are peer-governed institutions that put their own reputations on the line when they hire or promote researchers or publish research results. Indeed, both sets of intermediaries have stepped forward in recent years to scrutinize research for counterproductive financial incentives as well as for data fabrication, plagiarism, and other scientific misconduct.

Universities could be effective reputational intermediaries for biomedical researchers, and progress in this direction is being made. As discussed above, institutional compliance has the advantage of allowing clear relational obligations of employee to employer (rather than abstract duties to society or science) to define conflicts of interest, while centering public regulatory compliance at the institutional level where enforcement tends to be more straightforward (Sage 1997). Government's primary role in this framework would be to regulate institutional practices to further public goals regarding research ethics and productivity in the light of the service, research, and educational missions of nonprofit biomedical institutions.

This is a challenging assignment, notwithstanding the current extent of government oversight of research funding and administration. Industry represents a useful source of financial subsidy that supplements government funding of research, allows academic centers to offer salaries to clinical faculty that are competitive with private practice, and provides resources for education that relieve pressure on medical student tuition and graduate trainee stipends and working conditions. In addition, considerations of academic freedom limit, for good reasons, government's enforcement of research conduct and communication within universities.

Peer-reviewed medical journals could also be effective self-regulatory organizations to monitor financial flows in research, because they publish nearly all research findings and can make or break academic careers. The top journals such as the *New England Journal of Medicine* and *JAMA* (the *Journal of the American Medical Association*) wield enormous influence over public and professional opinion and generate huge windfalls in revenue and reputation for the professional associations that own them.

The editors of major medical journals have become exquisitely sensitive to actual and perceived impropriety, such as accepting paid advertising from pharmaceutical companies and publishing "editorials" authored by company consultants (Winker et al. 2000; Drazen and Curfman 2002; Gottlieb 2002; Hyman 2007). Most journals require disclosure to the editors of authors' funding and financial relationships for all articles, including the scientific submissions that are the journals' bread and butter, and in many cases the journals publish the disclosed information if and when the article appears in print. As with academic health centers (though, again, subject to constitutional and prudential considerations regarding freedom of speech and of the press), government could explicitly define the regulatory responsibilities of medical journals, which tend to be owned by nonprofit entities.

An explicitly regulatory orientation could also help improve the operation of institutional review boards (IRBs), the principal self-regulatory bodies charged with protecting human subjects within research institutions. IRBs are permanently embedded in the regulatory fabric of federal research but have come under criticism for being arbitrary and ineffectual (Hamburger 2004; Hyman 2007). One problem with IRBs is that their mission has been defined implicitly in relational terms—"representing" the interests of research participants—when their skills are often better suited to promoting transparency in research, ensuring that benefits to society justify particular studies, and protecting participants from unnecessary or excessive risks of harm.

The Flow of Information

Disclosure of information is a mainstay of relational governance. Short of outright prohibition, conflicts of interest are typically addressed by requiring agents to disclose competing demands to principal parties. The idea is that a principal with full information can decide whether or not to engage the agent, on what terms, and with what additional monitoring of performance. Disclosure requirements are often the first resort of policymakers concerned about conflicts of interest; several states and the federal government, for example, are considering publishing lists of doctors who accept gifts from drug companies.

Disclosure of conflicts of interest, however, is effective only if it is understandable. Framing researchers' financial incentives "objectively" for approval or rejection by research participants is challenging, given participants' varying degrees of education, cultural familiarity, and cognitive bias when presented with risks. To some research participants, financial incentives for researchers will seem corrupting, while others may believe that researchers with a financial stake in success will do a better job. Finally, disclosure is an imperfect solution to conflicts of interest if the agent making the disclosure already occupies a position of control and influence over the principal party (Sage 1999b).

Information policy based on public concerns is easier to design. Freed from the need to identify and cater to a principal party, regulation of research information can channel disclosure to audiences that can use it effectively, even if those are not the research participants themselves. Peer reviewers for journals, for example, may be a useful audience for required disclosure in connection with the review process. Because one manages what one measures, moreover, the research community can learn from examining its own practices with a view to disclosing them. Thus, a regulatory approach to transparency can emphasize information that promotes sound research when conveyed to health care providers and the public, rather than focusing only on how risks are communicated to participants.

Deemphasizing conflicts of interest as the justification for disclosure may even make information intended for research participants more useful to them. It may be possible to develop an intermediate form of disclosure that captures information of interest to research participants in a consistent, cost-effective form that can also be used by regulators. Mandatory disclosure by corporations issuing securities to the public, for example, is directed toward an identifiable group of likely investors but is also designed for use by government itself during pre-offering review of marketing materials. In health care, well-designed clinical trials registries might similarly serve this dual function.

Remedies for Injuries to Research Participants

A contradiction in the current federal approach to human subjects protection is that seemingly strong statements of concern for the welfare of research participants are not matched by individual recourse under federal law for injuries suffered in the course of research. Furthermore, unlike other countries, the United States does not require research institutions to have clinical trials insurance, and compensation policies for research injuries are erratic and incomplete (Steinbrook 2006).

Adhering to relational standards for judging conflicts of interest increases the risk of high-stakes litigation in today's financially charged research environment, forcing the debate over individual recourse into an all-or-nothing choice rather than a reasonable middle ground. In contrast, regulating financial flows as incentives serving public objectives would allow limited but meaningful individual remedies in the event of research injury. False or incomplete disclosure to human subjects of material facts about research risks—not about arguable sources of disloyalty—would give rise to legal claims for lack of informed consent or, in extreme cases, fraud. At the same time, abandoning a relational, fiduciary standard could avoid litigation where the causal link between the communications failure and the injury was attenuated. A useful analogy is whether liability for failing to obtain informed consent to treatment should include nondisclosure by physicians of their own financial incentives. Allowing claims for any injury received during medical care, because some fact about the financial structure of care was not discussed with the patient, substitutes open-ended liability for liability that arose under established informed-consent law only if an undisclosed physical risk of treatment manifested itself and caused harm.

Humanity and Compassion

One of the biggest public policy challenges in health care is preserving the "personal touch" in an increasingly specialized, industrialized, expensive, and bureaucratic system. Somewhat paradoxically, Anglo-American bioethics as translated into law has undercut the humanity of medical relationships (Hyman 1990; Sage 2001). The generation of bioethics captured in the "common rule" elevates patients' autonomy over professional beneficence. Some physicians have interpreted this preference as license to abdicate personal responsibility for their patients' welfare in favor of giving patients information and freedom of choice. Relational analysis of conflicts of interest carries this trend further by attaching legal consequences to any personal commitment by the agent other than to an identified principal party.

The current wave of attempts to ban contact between pharmaceutical company representatives and physicians, particularly trainees in academic medical centers, demonstrates the risks of this approach. Unlike previous conflict-of-interest policies, which emphasized the threat to professional judgment created by lavish gifts of cash or luxury goods from drug companies, the most recent prohibitions apply equally to token gestures that previously would have been considered harmless. Brennan and colleagues (2006), for example, argue that even small gifts will compromise physicians' decision-making by triggering social norms of reciprocity associated with the receipt of gifts, regardless of monetary value. They assert that banning those gifts and other opportunities for drug sales representatives to form friendships with physicians, such as industry-sponsored continuing medical education seminars, will make physicians dispassionate prescribers. In other words, industry critics seek to sever the human bond between physician and pharmaceutical representative in the name of strengthening the bond between physician and patient.

Can one dictate "caring" so selectively? Or does reducing human connection in one area reduce it in others? Physicians are not otherwise cloistered, nor should they be. For them and other health professionals—including, one would hope, biomedical researchers engaged in human subjects research—human impulses such as compassion and fellowship are indispensable. Moreover, a sense of personal solidarity with one's colleagues is considered to be at the heart of many professions. Would critics of pharmaceutical industry contacts reach consensus so easily if the question were whether physicians should recommend minimal-benefit, high-cost treatments because their personal relationship with a patient or family biased them to action rather than inaction, or whether physicians should socialize with other physicians and health professionals to whom they might refer patients?

It is true that drug detailers, like all accomplished salespeople, are trained to feign friendship to promote their products (Fugh-Berman and Ahari 2007). American health care, the world's most expensive cottage industry, is frighteningly susceptible not only to these blandishments but also to habitual practices and norms of behavior that have little scientific basis and enormous cost implications. The sunshine of disclosure is therefore salutary if it shames both physicians and medical suppliers into curtailing morally questionable practices. Still, walling off physicians from personal relationships with pharmaceutical representatives and other businesspeople, while hoping they deal humanely with patients, colleagues, and the needs of society, may prove impossible.

Explicit Relational Strictures for Some Research

Draining financial relationships of knee-jerk moral opprobrium in debates over the public duties of researchers creates opportunities for reinforcing fiduciary constructs in circumstances where they remain appropriate. That academic centers, as agents, serve many principals with different interests, for example, deserves greater public attention than it now receives. Academic health centers are supposed to balance patient care, research, and education, and they survive on a combination of revenue sources, including health insurance reimbursements, charitable contributions, public research grants, and industry contracts. Institutional conflict-of-interest policies for academic health centers need to provide not only transparency but also an explanation of these mixed missions to the public and private constituencies that rely on them.

Some institutional processes may require stricter safeguards. If IRBs enforcing regulatory standards no longer need consider themselves primarily agents for research participants, it may be advisable, in riskier studies, to appoint formal "research advocates" to represent individual participants, as Dresser (2003) proposes. Another possibility is to create external testing bodies for some new drugs and medical devices that are formally chartered as "public research auditors" (Pronovost, Miller, and Wachter 2007). Unlike academic health centers, these entities could be regulated in terms analogous to those applied to financial auditors, such as prohibitions on receiving payment in stock and on allowing inventors to direct the testing of their own products.

There is also a need to revisit the loyalty obligations of the treating physician to his or her patient in the research context. Physicians have never been "pure advocates" for patients, despite political desire, at the height of managed care, to charge them with this duty. Nonetheless, the law generally holds physicians to relational standards for representing their patients' interests. Coleman (2005) observes that the research physician's obligations to the participant as patient are in tension with good research practice at several points: randomization, standardized rather than customized treatment, data-gathering that offers no clinical benefit, and blinded study design, which can make it difficult to evaluate and respond to unexpected events. It is particularly hard to address conflicts of interest for physicians in solo or small-group clinical practice, whose main job is to help patients rather than to assist research and for whom a few thousand dollars in supplemental research payments can be a significant motivator.

Finder's fees paid to community physicians by clinical trials sites, mainly hospitals, in exchange for referring patients are an example of relational conflicts of interest (Lemmens and Miller 2003). Physicians owe direct fiduciary obligations to patients, and payment by a third party that is contingent on patients' participating in a specific research study will almost certainly influence the course of treatment that the physician recommends. In its barest form, a finder's fee for research recruitment is simply a kickback, no different than a side payment for prescribing a drug or admitting a patient to a hospital (American Medical Association 2006, 164).

Medicine has taken a surprisingly long time to recognize and respond to the conflict of interest inherent in these payments (Sage 1999a). Medical ethics has been more concerned with "free money" than with money paid by outside sources for actual work that physicians perform, such as research administration. Accordingly, the American Medical Association's (AMA's) first opinion on conflicts of interest in research (2006, 151, 185–86) required merely that "remuneration received by the researcher . . . be commensurate with the efforts of the researcher on behalf of the company." This rule had the unintended consequence of favoring payments to physicians who work really hard to get their patients to participate in studies—with a much higher attendant likelihood that the patient's original course of care will be altered as a result—over payments to physicians who maintain a passive but perhaps less harmful attitude. The AMA finally addressed this concern in a code revision, stating bluntly that "offering or accepting payment for referring patients to research studies (finder's fees) is unethical" (American Medical Association 2006, 166).

Even with this clarification, there is as yet no effective legal model for policing conflicts of interest for self-employed physicians who receive payment for assisting community-based research. The community setting is remote from most existing legal enforcement mechanisms. Medical licensing bodies concentrate their limited resources on extreme incompetence and criminality. Physicians are for-profit businesspeople, not subject to the state and federal nonprofit corporation and tax-exemption rules that apply to universities and community hospitals. As a result, the AMA's ethics opinions on research payments have yet to alter professional norms, and finder's fees and other recruitment incentives for physicians remain common. IRBs, which play the most important oversight role in the research regulatory system as currently constituted, are primarily concerned with activities within academic medical centers. Based on recent reports, moreover, the effectiveness of IRBs associated with for-profit contract research organizations is questionable (U.S. Government Accountability Office 2009). Consequently, IRBs can help avert flagrant community-based abuses of patient welfare but probably cannot articulate a vision of conflict management that has widespread application.

This gap in public policy will only prove more challenging in the future, because the National Institutes of Health's new clinical and translational roadmap calls for networks of community physicians who can recruit current patients as human subjects (Zerhouni and Alving 2006). It is doubtful, for example, that the AMA's revisionist bright-line prohibition on finder's fees will survive the emergence of electronically linked community physicians participating in government-sponsored research, as opposed to pharmaceutical company consultancies that were intended more to build prescribing goodwill than to generate scientific research.

A possible compromise is some combination of nonrelational federal regulation of research incentives, relational state regulation of physicians' financial arrangements, and individual litigation in state court in cases involving flagrant violations of fiduciary duty. At a minimum, informed consent requires that the treating physician disclose the uncertainties associated with the care he or she recommends, if it includes a research component. Disclosure of any specific financial interests a physician has in potential biomedical advances is probably warranted as well (American Medical Association 2004, 181).

Conclusion

As the biomedical research enterprise expands and restructures, many critics have been quick to condemn instances of money changing hands between researchers and other parties as "conflicts of interest." Criticism has also extended to nonfinancial incentives that, in the critics' opinion, might compromise what they consider fundamental values of biomedical research. In response to real instances of dishonest or sloppy research, some causing serious harm to patients or research participants, public and professional bodies have employed these "conflict-of-interest" arguments to require disclosure of many types of financial relationship and to suggest banning others. However, there is as yet no evidence that these reforms will be beneficial and little if any indication of how society might measure their effects.

Approaching the financing of research in this fashion is likely to fail, because it confuses researchers' obligations to specific parties such as research participants or academic employers ("relational duties") with their obligations to society as a whole ("regulatory duties"). The relational-regulatory balance in U.S. medicine is unstable, and the size of the U.S. health care system and the biomedical research enterprise it supports makes addressing that instability a priority for public policy.

Like many regulatory issues involving professions, conflict-of-interest policy in biomedical research is largely about change and resistance to change. Alleging conflict of interest is a common strategy for defenders of traditional practices. The superior alternative is to deal with financial flows as an overall question of research integrity and productivity, even if older generations of biomedical scientists are uncomfortable with the transformation of their work from a profession to a regulated industry.

By exploring relational and regulatory duties in the context of biomedical research, we can address the larger question of building a system of public accountability on a foundation of relational governance. Problems of relational-regulatory balance are not limited to biomedical research, nor even to health care. They arise frequently in rapidly industrializing sectors of the economy where private legal disputes governed by courts have been liberally supplemented, if not fully superseded, by public legislation and administrative law. Experience with conflicts of interest and incentives in these areas demonstrates the limits of using relational duties to serve broader social interests, as well as the need for carefully calibrated, empirically justifiable regulation.

Whether American society relies primarily on a system of relational research ethics (including conflicts of interest) or on a system of regulated research ethics (with fewer conflicts of interest) is a matter of substance, not merely semantics. The public duties incumbent upon ethical research have societal rather than individual benefits and therefore are not amenable to the usual control mechanisms for conflicts of interest. In other words, conflict-of-interest analysis cannot create the correct incentives to serve "principles" when those goals are not embodied in discrete, identifiable "principals."

ACKNOWLEDGMENT

An earlier version of this chapter was published as W. M. Sage, "Some Principles Require Principals: Why Banning 'Conflicts of Interest' Won't Solve Incentive Problems in Biomedical Research," *Texas Law Review* 85 (2007): 1412–63.

REFERENCES

AAMC Task Force on Financial Conflicts of Interest in Clinical Research. 2002. *Protecting Subjects, Preserving Trust, Promoting Progress II: Principles and Recommendations for Oversight of an Institution's Financial Interests in Human Subjects Research.* Washington, DC: Association of American Medical Colleges.

American Bar Association. 2007. *Model Rules of Professional Conduct.* Chicago: American Bar Association.

American Medical Association. 2004. *Code of Medical Ethics: Current Opinions with Annotations.* Chicago: American Medical Association.

———. 2006. *Code of Medical Ethics: Current Opinions with Annotations.* Chicago: American Medical Association.

Appelbaum, P. S. 2002. Clarifying the ethics of clinical research: A path toward avoiding the therapeutic misconception. *American Journal of Bioethics* 2 (2): 22–23.

Armstrong, D. 2005. Delicate operation: How a famed hospital invests in device it uses and promotes. *Wall Street Journal,* Dec. 12.

Association of American Medical Colleges. 2008. *Report of the AAMC Task Force on Industry Funding of Medical Education to the AAMC Executive Council, for Consideration, June 18–19.* Washington, DC: Association of American Medical Colleges.

Barnes, M., and P. S. Florencio. 2002. Investigator, IRB and institutional financial conflicts of interest in human-subjects research: Past, present, and future. *Seton Hall Law Review* 32:525–61.

Belsky, L., and E. J. Emanuel. 2004. Conflicts of interest and preserving the objectivity of scientific research. *Health Affairs* 23 (1): 268–70.

Brennan, T. A., D. J. Rothman, L. Blank, D. Blumenthal, S. C. Chimonas, J. J. Cohen, J. Goldman, et al. 2006. Health industry practices that create conflicts of interest. *JAMA* 295 (4): 429–33.

Coffee, J. C., Jr. 2004. Gatekeeper failure and reform: The challenge of fashioning relevant reforms. *Boston University Law Review* 84 (2): 301–64.

Coleman, C. H. 2005. Duties to subjects in clinical research. *Vanderbilt Law Review* 287 (2): 387–449.

Drazen, J. M., and G. D. Curfman 2002. Financial associations of authors. *New England Journal of Medicine* 346 (24): 1901–2.

Dresser, R. 2003. Patient advocates in research: New possibilities, new problems. *Washington University Journal of Law and Policy* 11:237–48.

DuVal, G. 2004. Institutional conflicts of interest: Protecting human subjects, scientific integrity, and institutional accountability. *Journal of Law, Medicine, and Ethics* 32 (4): 613–25.

Emanuel, E. J. 2004. Ending concerns about undue inducement. *Journal of Law, Medicine, and Ethics* 32 (1): 100–105.

Epstein, R. A. 1992. The legal regulation of lawyers' conflicts of interest. *Fordham Law Review* 60 (4): 579–93.

Fugh-Berman, A., and S. Ahari. 2007. Following the script: How drug reps make friends and influence doctors. *PLoS Medicine* 4 (4): e105. http://medicine.plosjournals.org.

Gottlieb, S. 2002. *New England Journal* loosens its rules on conflicts of interest. *BMJ* 324 (7352): 1474.

Hamburger, P. 2004. The new censorship: Institutional review boards. *Supreme Court Review*, 271–354.

Haskell, P. G. 1998. *Why Lawyers Behave as They Do.* Boulder, CO: Westview Press.

Hyman, D. A. 1990. How law killed ethics. *Perspectives in Biology and Medicine* 34 (1): 134–51.

———. 2007. Institutional review boards: Is this the least worst we can do? *Northwestern Law Review* 101 (2): 749–74.

Korn, D. 1996. Reengineering academic medical centers: Reengineering academic values? *Academic Medicine* 71 (10): 1033–43.

Koski, G. 2003. Research, regulations, and responsibility: Confronting the compliance myth: A reaction to Professor Gatter. *Emory Law Journal* 52 (1): 403–16.

Krimsky, S. 2003. *Science in the Private Interest: Has the Lure of Profits Corrupted Biomedical Research?* Lanham, MD: Rowman & Littlefield.

Lemmens, T., and P. B. Miller. 2003. The human subjects trade: Ethical and legal issues surrounding recruitment incentives. *Journal of Law, Medicine, and Ethics* 31 (3): 398–418.

Levinsky, N. G. 2002. Nonfinancial conflicts of interest in research. *New England Journal of Medicine* 347 (10): 759–61.

Meier, B. 2004. Contracts keep drug research out of reach. *New York Times*, Nov. 29.

Pronovost, P. J., M. Miller, and R. M. Wachter. 2007. The GAAP in quality measurement and reporting. *JAMA* 298 (15): 1800–1802.

Rennie, D. 1997. Thyroid storm. *JAMA* 277 (15): 1238–43.

Sage, W. M. 1997. Enterprise liability and the emerging managed health care system. *Law and Contemporary Problems* 60 (2): 159–210.

———. 1999a. Physicians as advocates. *Houston Law Review* 73 (5): 1529–1630.

———. 1999b. Regulating through information: Disclosure laws and American health care. *Columbia Law Review* 99 (7): 1701–1829.

———. 2001. The lawyerization of medicine. *Journal of Health Politics, Policy, and Law* 26 (5): 1179–95.

———. 2007a. Paying research subjects: The U.S. example. In *Essais cliniques, quels risques?* ed. A. Laude and D. Tabuteau. Paris: Presses Universitaires de France.

———. 2007b. Some principles require principals: Why banning "conflicts of interest" won't solve incentive problems in biomedical research. *Texas Law Review* 85 (6): 1413–63.

Steinbrook, R. 2005. Financial conflicts of interest and the Food and Drug Administration's advisory committees. *New England Journal of Medicine* 353 (2): 116–18.

———. 2006. Compensation for injured research subjects. *New England Journal of Medicine* 354 (18): 1871–73.

Stolberg, S. G. 1999. F.D.A. officials fault Penn team in gene therapy death. *New York Times,* Dec. 9.

Thompson, D. F. 1993. Understanding financial conflicts of interest. *New England Journal of Medicine* 329 (8): 573–76.

University of Texas at Austin. 2007. General compliance training program. www.utexas.edu/ administration/oic/cts/cw126e/alt/page4.htm.

U.S. Government Accountability Office. 2009. *Human Subjects Research: Undercover Tests Show the Institutional Review Board System Is Vulnerable to Unethical Manipulation.* GAO-09-448T. Washington, DC: U.S. Government Accountability Office.

Wendel, W. B. 2003. The deep structure of conflicts of interest. *Georgetown Journal of Legal Ethics* 16 (2): 473–504.

Werhane, P., and J. Doering. 1997. Conflicts of interest and conflicts of commitment. In *Research Ethics: A Reader,* ed. D. Elliott and J. E. Stern. Hanover, NH: University Press of New England.

Winker, M. A., A. Flanagin, B. Chi-Lum, J. White, K. Andrews, R. L. Kennett, C. D. DeAngelis, and R. A. Musacchio. 2000. Guidelines for medical and health information sites on the Internet: Principles governing AMA websites. *JAMA* 283 (12): 1600–1606.

Zerhouni, E. A., and B. Alving. 2006. Clinical and translational science award: A framework for a national research agenda. *Translational Research* 148 (1): 4–5.

PART III

MANAGEMENT TODAY
AND IN THE FUTURE

Current Regulations, Comparison of Guidelines, and Considerations for Policy Development

DAVID PERLMAN, PH.D.

With the increased attention to conflicts of interest by government agencies, Congress, professional societies, and the public, many academic institutions have developed or revised their policies, procedures, and practices for managing such conflicts. This chapter discusses the current regulatory regime and ethical, policy, and operational considerations that institutions might wish to consider when developing or revising policies to manage financial conflicts of interest in biomedical research. I highlight some of the recent events that have prompted increased scrutiny in the area of conflicts of interest and how this increased scrutiny affects compliance efforts and public trust in the research enterprise. To assist institutions in undertaking the task of revising or developing conflict-of-interest policies and procedures in the light of recent reports and guidance documents, I provide a detailed comparison of the current regulations to several of these reports and guidance documents. Such a comparison could help institutions consider several key policy elements that will help bolster public trust in the research enterprise through proactive and effective management of financial conflicts of interest.

Financial conflicts of interest in biomedical research have received significant attention from numerous key sectors in recent years. Several high-profile cases have brought to the fore concerns about conflicts of financial interests held by investigators and the institutions that sponsor or support research. Two cases, in particular, featured a combination of investigators' and institutions' financial interests. The first case involved a gene transfer investigator, at a major health sciences university, who had licensed the vector used in human studies to a private company. The investigator and the institution held significant financial interests in the company, involving equity positions and options, should the vector become a commercial success (Drug Information Association 2004). The second case involved a well-known cancer center and investigators who held equity interests in a product under investigation at the center (Nelson 2001). The equity interests in both cases exceeded the current Food and Drug Administration (FDA) levels for acceptable financial interests held by clinical investigators.

Partly as a result of such cases, numerous professional and industry associations, as well as Congress and other government bodies—including the U.S. General Accounting Office (2001) and the now defunct National Bioethics Advisory Commission (2001)—became concerned that financial conflicts of interest might compromise the integrity of the scientific research enterprise and the investigators and institutions involved in it. In the past few years, several prominent organizations, including the Association of American Medical Colleges (AAMC) (AAMC Taskforce on Financial Conflicts of Interest in Clinical Research 2001, 2002), the Association of American Universities (AAU) (2002), the American Medical Association (AMA) (Morin et al. 2002), the American College of Physicians and American Society of Internal Medicine (Coyle 2002a, 2002b), the International Committee of Medical Journal Editors (2001), the Pharmaceutical Research and Manufacturers of America (2002), and many others, have issued reports or policy recommendations related to conflicts of interest in the biomedical sciences.

The increased attention and concern over conflicts of interest has sparked several responses. At last count, various professional societies or government bodies have released more than ten reports, with specific recommendations for addressing, managing, or eliminating conflicts of financial interests held by investigators and the institutions that sponsor or support research. Congressional concerns have led to issuance of draft interim (2001) and final interim (2003) guidance from the FDA and the Office of Human Research Protections, the two government agencies responsible for the regulation and conduct of clinical research in the United States (U.S. Department of Health and Human Services 2001, 2003). Articles from the popular press suggest to the public that existing protections for human subjects who volunteer to participate in research are not adequate or that gains from research—in terms of money, prestige, publications, and honors—are more important to investigators and their institutions than preserving the safety of human subjects (Gillis 2002; Lemonick and Goldstein 2002).

While new regulations are not anticipated, taken together, the numerous reports and guidance documents released in the past few years have produced corresponding fears from research administrators, senior officials at academic medical centers, and pharmaceutical company executives. All of these stakeholders are (or ought to be) concerned that existing conflict-of-interest management systems are inadequate or will require significant investment in terms of personnel, resources, space, and procedural changes to meet what surely will become "best-practice" standards for measuring these management processes. Institutions, then, should begin examining their current policies, practices, and systems to determine what changes or investments should be made to ensure their conflict-of-interest management systems are "up to spec." As an address by bioethicist Arthur Caplan suggested, failure to have in place adequate systems for monitoring conflicts of interest of investigators and institutions represents a weakening of one of the core protections for human subjects in the current regulatory regime (Drug Information Association 2004). To assist in this charge, I attempt here to distill the recommendations from the reports and guidance documents in the light of current regulations for managing conflicts of interest, for those who will be called on to assess their conflict-of-interest management systems.

Financial Conflicts of Interest and Public Trust in the Research Enterprise

"Conflict of interest" can be defined as any situation in which financial or personal obligations may compromise or present the appearance of compromising an investigator's professional judgment in conducting or reporting research (Russell-Einhorn and Puglisi 2001).[1] Individual investigators' financial interests can take many forms. They can be straightforward, such as consulting fees, stock ownership, honoraria, or salary from entities with a role in the research. Alternatively, they may include more subtle interests, such as intellectual property rights, financial incentives offered by pharmaceutical or biotechnology companies to researchers or physicians for conducting trials or enrollment of subjects, or financial relationships from spousal employment.

Institutional financial interests are a separate, but related, matter. An institutional financial interest occurs when either the institution itself or one of its senior officials with research-related decision-making responsibilities holds significant financial interests in companies or technologies under study at the institution or in intellectual property licensed from its faculty to private companies. Institutional financial interests include the interests of senior officials, because these officials frequently have decision-making responsibilities that can significantly influence research funding and resources at the institution. Any of these financial incentives—whether held by an individual investigator, the institution that supports or funds the research, or both—may adversely affect the collection, analysis, and interpretation of data, scientific objectivity and integrity, and, ultimately, public trust in the research enterprise (AAMC Taskforce 2002).

Regardless of the source of funding for research, the public, whose members will be recruited to volunteer to test drugs, devices, and other investigational agents, must be assured that their interests and welfare will be protected to the fullest extent possible. The principle of justice, as articulated in the Belmont Report (National Commission for the Protection of Human Subjects in Biomedical and Behavioral Research 1979), which espouses ethical principles central to protecting human subjects, demands that the benefits and the burdens of research be distributed equitably. Numerous examples of past research ethics abuses, such as the Public Health Service sponsorship of the "Tuskegee Study of Untreated Syphilis in the Negro Male" and radiation experiments sponsored by various agencies of the U.S. government, when viewed collectively, have damaged the public's trust in the research enterprise by violating the ethical principles in the Belmont Report. More recently, as noted above, the realization that research investigators and research institutions involved in gene transfer research and other product-development research held significant equity interests in commercialization of the agents under study has intensified public concern regarding, and scrutiny of, the financial interests present in the research enterprise. Despite the diversity of financial, professional, and personal interests that might compromise scientific integrity and institutional and personal commitments to protect human subjects, current regulatory requirements for conflicts of interest in the biomedical sciences address only a small subset of these interests.

Current Regulations

Three different sets of regulations address financial conflicts of interest in biomedical research. One set, promulgated by the U.S. Public Health Service

(PHS), addresses how *institutions* should handle individual investigators' financial conflicts of interest. A second set governs *individual* investigators' disclosure of financial conflicts of interest to sponsors of research regulated by the FDA. Finally, regulations for the protection of human subjects in research raise the issue of conflicts of interest in research for members of institutional review boards (IRBs). The manner in which institutions address these regulatory requirements depends on the source of funding for the research.

> *PHS Regulations (1995).* Institutions receiving federal research funds from PHS agencies such as the National Institutes of Health (NIH) must comply with the PHS regulations at 42 Code of Federal Regulations (CFR) Part 50, Subpart F (U.S. Public Health Service 1995). These regulations require institutions to establish conflict-of-interest policies and procedures and appoint a conflict-of-interest official or committee to manage reporting of financial conflicts of interest from investigators and to appropriate agencies of the federal government.

> *FDA Regulations (1998).* If the institution conducts research involving FDA-regulated test articles, FDA regulations at 21 CFR Part 54 (U.S. Food and Drug Administration 1998) also require that investigators disclose information related to their financial interests to the research sponsor, so that the sponsor can inform the FDA. Ideally, the institution also should be notified about that disclosure.

> *IRB Regulations.* Regulations for the protection of human subjects in research at 45 CFR Sec. 46.107(e) (U.S. Department of Health and Human Services 1991) and 21 CFR Sec. 56.107(e) (U.S. Food and Drug Administration 1981) require that IRB members with conflicting interests refrain from participating in the voting and discussion of protocols, except to answer questions by the IRB. Certainly, an IRB member who has a financial stake in the approval of a protocol would be considered to have a conflict of interest.

Thus, an institution that receives funds from a PHS agency, conducts research on FDA-regulated test articles, and has an IRB must adhere to all these regulations. Tables 9.1, 9.2, and 9.3 provide additional details on these regulatory requirements.

There are two problems with the current regulations. First, while the IRB is charged with ensuring the protection of human subjects, it lacks a specific regulatory requirement for managing investigators' or institutions' conflicts of interest. As the AAMC Task Force on Financial Conflicts of Interest in Clin-

TABLE 9.1.
42 CFR Part 50, Subpart F, Applies to Institutions
Receiving Public Health Service Funding

Regulatory Considerations

1. Does the institution have policy in place that defines "significant financial interest"?
2. Does the institution have policy in place that describes the institution's responsibilities? Examples:
    a. Informing investigators of their responsibilities and the existence of 42 CFR Part 50, Subpart F.
    b. Designating an institutional official or committee to solicit and review financial disclosures.
    c. Establishing guidelines to identify, manage, reduce, or eliminate conflicts of interest and establishing enforcement mechanisms.

Source: U.S. Public Health Service 1995.

TABLE 9.2.
21 CFR Part 54 Applies to Investigators Conducting Research involving Food
and Drug Administration–Regulated Test Articles

Regulatory Considerations

1. Does the institution have policy in place that defines when investigators must disclose conflict-related information to the study sponsor?
2. Does the institution have policy in place that describes how frequently conflict-of-interest information should be updated with the sponsor?
3. As a best practice, is the institution notified when investigators disclose information to study sponsors?

Source: U.S. Food and Drug Administration 1998.

TABLE 9.3.
45 CFR Sec. 46.107(e) and 21 CFR Sec. 56.107(e) Apply If the Institution
Has an Institutional Review Board (IRB)

Regulatory Considerations

1. Does IRB policy state that no member may participate in initial or continuing review of research in which he or she has a conflicting interest, except to provide information requested by the IRB?
2. Does the IRB as a best practice document the recusal of IRB members with conflicting interests in the IRB meeting minutes?
3. Does IRB policy define (or provide procedures for determining) what might constitute a conflicting interest?

Sources: U.S. Department of Health and Human Services 1991; U.S. Food and Drug Administration 1981.

ical Research (2001, 5) concludes, "Current federal regulations concerning financial interests in research were intended to promote objectivity in federally-funded research and to ensure the reliability of data submitted to the FDA, not to protect human subjects *per se.*" Nevertheless, the regulatory authority of the IRB is broad, and many IRBs feel compelled to include consideration of conflicts of interest when reviewing research (U.S. General Accounting Office 2001). However, without regulations to guide them, IRBs might feel inadequate to meet the task. Many of the recent guidance documents produced by professional associations and the U.S. Department of Health and Human Services (DHHS) are specifically designed to address this "gap" in the system for protecting human subjects.

Second, the regulations that govern conflicts of interest concern only the interests of investigators. Financial interests of institutions or senior officials within such institutions are not addressed, despite numerous reports and guidance documents recently produced by professional associations indicating that such institutional conflicts of interest require greater scrutiny and pose an equal risk of undermining public trust in the research enterprise (AAMC Task Force 2002). As a result of these two problems with the current regulations, many institutions are realizing that their policies, procedures, and practices regarding management of financial conflicts of interest may need to be revised.

Comparison of Guidance Documents and Reports

Tables 9.4 and 9.5 provide detailed comparisons of two of the most widely cited reports on conflicts of interest and the recent DHHS guidance to assist institutions that are now examining their processes for managing such conflicts. I refer to these documents in discussing some implementation strategies and management decisions that research administrators and institutions should consider in developing effective conflict-of-interest management mechanisms.[2]

Table 9.4 compares two of these reports (Association of American Universities 2002 and AAMC Taskforce 2001; hereafter referred to as the AAU and AAMC reports) and one guidance document (U.S. Department of Health and Human Services 2003; hereafter referred to as DHHS guidance) on issues related to individual investigators' conflicts of interest. Table 9.5 does the same for institutional conflicts of interest.

Three specific and interrelated aspects of these documents are highlighted in the following discussions of individual and institutional conflicts of interest: the definition of "significant financial interest," disclosure requirements, and management of reported financial interests.

Individual Investigators' Conflicts of Interest
Defining "Significant Financial Interest"

The AAU and AAMC reports define "significant financial interest" in much the same way as the PHS definition at 42 CFR Part 50, Subpart F, with one or

TABLE 9.4.

Conflict-of-Interest Reports and Documents: Investigators' Conflicts of Interest (COIs)

Issue	AAMC	AAU	DHHS
Differences			
Definition of financial interest?	Similar to current PHS definition, including exclusions	Recommends a definition consistent with PHS and NSF definitions, including royalty interests	Anything of monetary value, such as payments for services, equity interests, or intellectual property
Definition of when a financial interest is (can be) a conflict?	Rebuttable presumption that any significant financial interest poses a conflict	When financial interests may (appear to) compromise investigator's professional judgment	When financial interest creates or may be reasonably expected to create a bias
Disclosure standard?	PHS *de minimis* standards	Disclose all interests ("zero tolerance" disclosure threshold) is one recommended practice	Not specifically addressed (presumably PHS and FDA standards are the thresholds)
Level of independence in COI process?	Independent monitoring (external to the institution) might be required	Not discussed for individual investigators' COIs, but discussed for institutional COIs	Independent monitoring (external to the institution); independent oversight of informed-consent process
Two-Point Similarities (in italics)			
Recommendations for IRB members' COIs?	*No*	*No*	Yes

Disclosure to others external to the institution?	*To journal editors, at oral presentations, to federal agencies, to research subjects (as required by IRB)*	*To journal editors, at oral presentations, to federal agencies, to research subjects (as required by IRB)*	Not addressed in detail
Rebuttable presumption and/or compelling circumstances?	*Yes*	Yes (although not articulated specifically using those terms)	No
Standards apply to all research regardless of funding?	*Yes*	*Yes*	No
COI review before IRB review?	*Yes*	*Yes*	Not specifically addressed
Three-Point Similarities			
Disclosure to whom at the institution?	COI committee with wide representation to IRB	COI committee with wide representation to IRB	COI committee with wide representation to IRB
Community representation on COI committee?	Recommended	Recommended	Recommended
COI process separate from IRB?	Yes	Yes	Yes
Level of transparency in COI process?	Internal reporting and external disclosure, as necessary	Internal reporting and external disclosure, as necessary	Internal reporting and external disclosure, as necessary

Note: AAMC refers to the report of the AAMC Task Force on Financial Conflicts of Interest in Clinical Research 2001; AAU, to the report of the Association of American Universities 2002; DHHS, to the report of the U.S. Department of Health and Human Services 2003.

Abbreviations: PHS, U.S. Public Health Service; NSF, National Science Foundation; FDA, U.S. Food and Drug Administration; IRB, institutional review board.

TABLE 9.5.

Conflict-of-Interest Reports and Documents: Institutional Conflicts of Interest (COIs)

Issue	AAMC	AAU	DHHS
Differences			
Definitions of institutional financial interest?	Institution receives royalties from investigational product; equity interest through technology transfer; *or* officer has significant financial interest in sponsor or product, including equity interest, consulting fees, honoraria, gifts, or certain appointments	Institution has interests involving equity or royalty arrangements in research programs, especially those where interest is derived from university technology transfers; *and* officials have the same interests as above	Anything of monetary value, such as payments for services, equity interests, or intellectual property
Categorization of who might hold such interests and thus who ought to report interests?	1. The institution 2. Its officers 3. IRB and COIC chairs and members	1. The institution 2. Its officers 3. Affiliated foundations	1. The institution 2. Its officers 3. Other interested parties
Technology transfer disclosure and/or reporting to COIC?	Yes	Disclosure not specifically discussed but should be considered	Disclosure not specifically discussed
Disclosure to others external to the institution?	Recommended disclosure to human subjects, in form determined by IRB; disclosure in publications	Not specifically discussed but should be considered	Not specifically discussed
Rebuttable presumption and/or compelling circumstances for interests when human subjects involved?	Yes	Standard for disclosure not robustly developed, but a standard should be developed	Standard for disclosure not robustly developed
Standards apply to all research regardless of funding?	Yes	Not specifically addressed	No
Two-Point Similarities (in italics)			
Management process outlined?	*Yes; if COIs cannot be eliminated through recusal or managed through appropriate procedures, research should not be conducted within or under auspices of the institution*	*Yes; disclose always; manage in most cases; prohibit interest when necessary to protect public or university interest*	*Not in any level of detail*

Institutional COIC separate and distinct from COIC for individual investigators' COIs?	*Recommended*	*Recommended*	Discussed but not specifically endorsed
Recusal of COIC members who have a COI?	Yes	*Not specifically addressed*	*Not specifically addressed*
Three-Point Similarities			
Definition of when an institutional financial interest is (can be) a conflict?	Whenever financial interests of the institution (or official) might (appear to) affect institutional processes for conduct, review, or oversight of research	When institution (or official) has an external relationship or financial interest in a faculty research project that can lead to bias	When financial interest creates or may be reasonably expected to create a bias
Disclose to COIC for institutional COIs?	Yes	Yes	Yes
Community representative on COIC?	Recommended	Recommended	Recommended
Disclosure to others at the institution?	To IRB	To IRB	To IRB
Level of independent monitoring in COI process?	Yes; when investigator or research official has COI in procurement process; when institution receives gifts from sponsor; when institution serves only as trial investigative site; independent IRB review recommended	Yes; an independent research-monitoring process is recommended to ensure that potential conflicts do not undermine the integrity of the work and the institution	Yes; recommends that independent organizations hold or administer the institution's financial interest
Firewall between research financial decisions and research approval decisions?	Yes	Yes	Yes

Note: AAMC refers to the report of the AAMC Task Force on Financial Conflicts of Interest in Clinical Research 2002; AAU, to the report of the Association of American Universities 2002; DHHS, to the report of the U.S. Department of Health and Human Services 2003.

Abbreviations: IRB, institutional review board; COIC, conflict-of-interest committee.

two small differences. For instance, the PHS regulations exclude royalty interests paid by the institution, whereas the AAMC report (2001, 13) includes all "royalty income or the right to receive future royalties under a patent license or copyright, where the research is directly related to the licensed technology or work." Institutions developing policies should be aware of these differences, because how specific institutions choose to define "significant financial interest" will have a direct impact on what investigators are required to disclose. Those institutions that conduct FDA-regulated research should also remember to include the FDA financial disclosure requirements at 21 CFR Part 54.

Once a significant financial interest is identified, the institution should define how it should be handled in its policies and procedures. PHS regulations allow institutions to manage financial interests even if an interest exceeds the defined thresholds. In general, institutions can follow two approaches when determining how best to manage the financial interests of investigators. The first assumes that all significant financial interests should be prohibited. According to this "zero tolerance" policy, if an investigator's disclosed financial interests exceed the thresholds, he or she should not be allowed to conduct the research unless the financial interest is reduced or eliminated. The second approach, referred to by the AAMC report as the "rebuttable presumption" against financial interests, assumes that all significant financial interests require close scrutiny and that an investigator must provide "compelling circumstances" to receive institutional approval to initiate research despite the presence of a particular financial interest. This approach does not focus solely on the existence of a financial interest itself; rather, it focuses on (1) whether the individual investigator who has a financial interest is crucial to the successful and ethical conduct of the research by dint of expertise or other factors, and (2) how the research can continue with appropriate oversight and management.

Disclosure Requirements and Management of Reported Interests

How an institution chooses to define "significant financial interest" will have a direct impact on investigators' disclosure requirements and how the institution handles those disclosures. Each report directly addresses these topics. For instance, while the AAU report endorses a definition of financial interest similar to that in the AAMC report, it recommends that institutions consider adopting the "zero tolerance" disclosure threshold, as noted above.

The rationale is that many financial interests are not conflicts, and given the complex nature of some financial arrangements, it is appropriate to disclose all interests and evaluate such interests, case by case. For instance, in an NIH report issued in 1999, a working group of institutions recommended that the PHS disclosure thresholds for equity interest (currently, $10,000 or 5% ownership interest) should vary, depending on institutionally determined circumstances (Mahoney 1999). While the DHHS has not allowed the thresholds to be changed, individual institutions have the option to establish lower thresholds than those mandated by current regulations. The advantage of this approach would be to allow the conflict-of-interest official or committee to review all financial interests without placing the burden on investigators to make a subjective judgment as to whether they have a financial interest that requires disclosure.

The current PHS regulations require that, at a minimum, institutions select an official to review conflict-of-interest disclosures and decide how to manage them. However, the best-practice recommendation from the AAU and AAMC reports and the DHHS guidance is that a conflict-of-interest committee with wide representation should review financial disclosures. Smaller institutions, which might lack both the human and the financial resources to establish a committee that must convene to review disclosures, might find it burdensome to achieve this recommended best practice. As an alternative, smaller institutions might choose to appoint an official and an "advisory" committee that would meet less frequently. The official would make provisional judgments on financial disclosures, and the committee would provide oversight through periodic reviews of the conflict-of-interest official's management decisions and would be available to the official for guidance and advice as needed. For institutions with committees, the recommended best practice in all of the reports is to include at least one external member with no ties to the institution to serve on the committee. This best practice is intended to increase the transparency of the process and thus bolster public trust in the institution and its investigators. Therefore, institutions that wish to be "beyond reproach" in terms of how they handle conflicts of interest should strongly consider adding unaffiliated persons to their conflict-of-interest committees and review process.

Another important aspect concerns feedback to the IRB regarding conflict-of-interest determinations. The AAMC, AAU, and DHHS all recommend that conflict-of-interest determinations be reported to the IRB for consideration in the board's review process.[3] Regarding how the IRB should be included in conflict-of-interest management decisions, the AAMC report (2001, 8) suggests that "between the COI [conflict-of-interest] committee and the IRB, the most stringent determination should be dispositive."

Finally, for significant financial interests, the AAMC and AAU reports recommend that disclosure be made to regulatory bodies as required by statute, to journal editors, to audience members before oral presentations, and, as required by the IRB, to human research participants during the informed-consent process.

Institutional Conflicts of Interest

With the introduction of the Bayh-Dole Act of 1980 to encourage licensing of publicly funded technologies and research innovations to private sector companies, individual innovators and institutions received a mandate to establish financial arrangements with private companies. The private sector has the capital, means of production, and marketing apparatus that universities usually lack, whereas universities have the pool of talented innovators working on complex research and technological problems that industry has traditionally lacked. In recent years, due largely to an increase in both the complexity and number of financial arrangements between investigators and private sponsors, institutions have organized administrative structures to manage technology transfer licensing, clinical trials agreements for individual investigators, and other industry-academic partnerships. Using this administrative model, all three parties stand to benefit financially. The institution owns the patent or license on behalf of the innovator, with financial rewards accruing to both parties, and the sponsor bringing the technology or research product to market reaps the economic rewards from a successful product launch into the marketplace. However, a lack of adequate checks and balances or regulations to guide institutions, together with severe budgetary and fiscal pressures and the competition for talent and reputation at institutions of higher education, can mean that the financial arrangements of many academic institutions create the same specter of actual or perceived financial conflicts of interest that has plagued clinical investigators.

Currently, no agency of the federal government regulates the financial arrangements of institutions with industry sponsors of research or technological innovation.[4] Several notable cases, as discussed earlier in the chapter, have brought the issue of an institution's financial interests to the fore. The AAU report and DHHS guidance on financial conflicts of interest address the issue, and the AAMC Taskforce has issued a separate report (2002) with pol-icy recommendations and considerations on how institutions should ethi-cally respond to their own financial interests in biomedical research involving human subjects.

The recommendations for institutional conflict-of-interest management are similar to those for individual conflicts of interest in several ways, as table 9.5 indicates. In addition, the AAMC and AAU reports recommend separa-tion of the management process and review committees for institutional and individual investigators' financial arrangements. In contrast, the DHHS guid-ance does not clearly endorse such separation. Other major differences be-tween these three reports include the following: the definition of institutional financial interest, disclosure of financial interests, and management of po-tential conflicts of interest.

Definition of Financial Interest

Both the AAMC and AAU reports distinguish financial interests in terms of the financial holdings of the institution itself (e.g., equity, royalty, or other investments) versus the financial holdings of or decisions made by officials of the institution. The AAMC report (2002, 6–7) provides five criteria for deter-mining whether an official has a significant financial interest and offers ad-ditional examples of situations that may help identify when an official holds a significant interest. While not exhaustive, these five criteria suggest areas that institutions should address in developing policies to manage institutional financial arrangements and conflicts of interest. Two notable areas include the institution's purchasing/procurement decision-making process and receipt of gifts and in-kind contributions. The latter example poses additional consider-ations for policy development, because it expands the scope of financial inter-ests to include philanthropic aspects. Such considerations suggest that institu-tions will require processes to appropriately distinguish gifts from sponsored program funds and to foster good communication and data-sharing between an institution's research administration and development functions.

Disclosure of Institutional Financial Interests

Both the AAMC and AAU reports recommend that institutional financial ar-rangements be disclosed to an institutional conflict-of-interest committee and to the IRB. The AAMC report further recommends that any institutional financial arrangements related to technology transfer be disclosed to the conflict-of-interest committee and that institutional conflicts of interest be disclosed to human subjects, as determined by the IRB, and to journal editors. The DHHS and AAU guidelines do not specifically discuss these additional disclosures.

Management of Potential Interests

If the institution determines that it has a significant financial interest, precisely how it manages that interest becomes a particularly sensitive issue. The institution must ensure that it maintains its responsibilities both to protect human subjects involved in the research and to protect public confidence in the integrity of academic research institutions. Failure to do so might result in negative public sentiment, decreased support for the institution itself, and increased public concern that might spark government efforts to regulate institutions' financial arrangements in research.

While identification of institutional conflicts of interest requires vigilance and diligence, the management of these identified interests becomes a litmus test for the institution's policies and procedures and for its ethical culture and public esteem. Therefore, as it relates to the financial interests of institutional officials, recusal from research-financing decisions is a common recommendation. However, recusal may not be possible in all situations. The AAMC report recommends that the institution apply the "rebuttable presumption" standard to the management of institutional conflicts of interest when human subjects are involved. But the report further recommends that if the conflict-of-interest review finds that both a significant conflict and compelling circumstances exist, additional review and oversight by an external body, independent of the institution, should be considered. Some institutions may choose to have the external body review the research and its associated financial arrangements first. This process would allow the external review body to make the sometimes difficult decision that the circumstances presented are not "compelling" enough to rebut the presumption against eliminating the financial interest.

In relation to multicenter clinical trials, the AAMC report recommends that an institution with a conflict of interest should not serve as the primary site for the trial or as the coordinating center, unless the conflict can be eliminated through recusal or other steps. Furthermore, both the AAU and AAMC reports endorse the use of an external monitoring body to monitor and closely scrutinize such trials "to ensure that potential conflicts do not undermine the integrity of the work (and of the university)" (AAMC Taskforce 2001, 14).

Other recommendations for management processes and/or plans for institutional conflicts of interest include an independent organization to hold or administer the institution's financial interests, as in the DHHS guidance, and development of "firewalls" between research financial and research approval decisions, as in the AAMC reports of 2001 and 2002 and the DHHS guidance. Firewalls between the management of financial investments or endowments, human subjects protection, and technology transfer functions, through either organizational structure or management responsibilities, ensure greater balance in institutional decision-making. Each function, while supporting the mission of the institution, has different goals, all of which may conflict. Management of financial investments seeks opportunities to increase the financial strength of the institution through investment returns, including equity. Technology transfer seeks partnerships with industry that foster development of institutional technologies in the commercial marketplace. Human subject protection programs seek well-designed research protocols that adhere to the principles of the Belmont Report and the DHHS and FDA human subjects requirements. Policy must therefore ensure that (1) these different functions are sufficiently segregated so that their structure, composition, and activities do not foster, in themselves, an institutional conflict of interest; and (2) these functions are sufficiently independent from one another to ensure appropriate due diligence efforts in cases where institutional financial interests are present. Institutions should thus examine organizational and reporting lines, as well as processes developed to manage institutional conflicts of interest, when developing their policies and procedures in this area.

Management Decisions

Having discussed many aspects of similarity and divergence between the AAU and AAMC reports and recent federal guidance on both investigators' and institutions' financial conflicts of interest, I now turn to actual decisions that institutions or those charged with management of financial conflicts of interest might make in developing or revising their own policies on these subjects.

Step One. Institutions should ensure that their systems and policies and procedures are compliant with applicable regulations (FDA, PHS, and/ or IRB regulations). Tables 9.1, 9.2, and 9.3 provide guidance for assessing compliance with financial conflict-of-interest regulations.
Step Two. Institutions interested in proactively developing systems and

policies and procedures that exceed the current regulations should develop an institutional plan for managing, first, individual investigators' and then the institution's financial conflicts of interest. In the plan, institutions should be sure to address several conflict-of-interest management decisions. The remainder of the chapter discusses these decisions and what considerations might drive them.

Who and What Should Be Covered by the Conflict-of-Interest Policy?

Given the dual focus of the recent guidance and reports, an institution may wish to cover all individuals involved in research, in addition to clinical investigators, in its conflict-of-interest policy. Which parties to cover depends on the types of research the institution conducts or sponsors. For example, clinical trials of FDA-regulated test articles, regardless of the source of sponsorship—commercial or investigator-initiated—must comply with FDA regulations at 21 CFR Part 54. Cooperative oncology trials involving the National Cancer Institute must comply with the PHS regulations, because these trials involve funding support from a federal agency. Basic science and translational research may or may not be covered by conflict-of-interest regulation, but given the trend toward faculty-initiated basic science research, followed by faculty-initiated technology transfer or commercial spin-offs, institutions should consider including all types of research in their conflict-of-interest policies.

Another important question is what threshold for reporting financial interests should be used when the institution has multiple reporting responsibilities. This consideration is important because FDA and PHS regulations have different disclosure thresholds and different definitions of what constitutes a financial interest or a conflict of interest. For the sake of simplicity, and in accordance with the distilled recommendations of the recent guidance and reports, institutions might choose to adapt a single disclosure threshold.

Conflict-of-Interest Official or Committee?

Institutions need to decide whether one individual, an entire committee, or some combination of the two should be responsible for managing conflicts of interest. There are several factors to consider in making this decision: (1) institutional size, including the number of investigators, the volume of research conducted, and institutional resources; (2) the potential review, investigation, and management workload; and (3) whether the institutional culture is such that diversity of input is valued or involvement from major constituencies at the institution is required to implement important management decisions. For instance, as indicated earlier in the chapter, institutions may wish to have an advisory committee that allows the conflict-of-interest official to make expedited, noncontroversial decisions according to set policy or protocol.

When Does an Interest Create a Conflict, and How Should Such Conflicts Be Managed?

Although the disclosure thresholds and types of financial interest are well defined, PHS regulations give institutions wide latitude in determining how conflicts are managed once an interest reaches the level of a conflict of interest. Institutions must decide how they will manage actual and perceived conflicts of interest that might damage the institution's reputation.

The answer to the question of what standard the institution should choose to handle disclosure of financial interests can have a great impact on how financial conflicts of interest are managed at the institution. If the institution decides to implement the "rebuttable presumption" and "compelling circumstances" standards articulated in the AAMC report, it might more easily manage, up-front, any potential threats to institutional integrity. Institutions interested in complete proactive management might choose to implement an even stricter, "zero tolerance" standard, by which all entities covered by the institution's policy would make disclosures of all financial interests, and the conflict-of-interest official or committee would determine which interests constituted conflicts of interest and how to manage those conflicts.

Some Examples of How to Manage Conflicts of Interest

While not exhaustive, the following list contains examples of how institutions might choose to manage particular financial conflicts of interest.

- Public disclosure of the financial interests
- Monitoring of the research by independent reviewers
- Modification of the research plan
- Complete divestiture of interests from the research sponsor, product, or entity under study or considered for potential commercial development and/or licensing

- Selection of another investigator or research staff member to serve as the principal investigator
- Disclosure of the conflicting interest in the informed-consent document and/or any manuscripts or oral presentations relating to the research or product in question
- Severance of relationships that create actual or potential conflicts

To Whom Should Disclosures Be Made?

Several of the methods to manage or eliminate financial conflicts of interest concern disclosure. The question then becomes to whom such disclosures should be made.

PHS regulations require that individual investigators disclose their financial interests to the institution. It is then a question of whether an institution, which might have significant financial holdings of its own, is in the best position to judge which of its own interests might pose a conflict.

IRB regulations require that IRB members be free from conflicting interests in reviewing research. However, there is little guidance on what might constitute a conflicting interest, which leads to the question of whether the IRB can fairly determine the conflicts of its own members.

If part of the management of a conflict entails disclosure to research participants in the informed-consent document or during the informed-consent process, would research participants know what to make of such disclosures, whether they concern the individual investigator or the institution? The answer would depend, in part, on both the disclosure and how the participant understands it. Some participants might view with distrust a disclosure that an investigator or institution stands to benefit financially from the research in which they participate. Alternatively, some participants might equate, however unwittingly and incorrectly, a financial interest in the product under study with expertise on the part of the investigator. The danger of misunderstanding of the research process or of potential therapeutic misconception on the part of participants (Appelbaum et al. 1987) cannot be dismissed, unless the investigator is careful to distinguish between the research and the financial interest in the product under study. Moreover, if an adequate and proper informed-consent process is not followed, the danger of therapeutic misrepresentation might further complicate matters (McCluskey 2002).

FDA regulations require that investigators disclose financial interests to the sponsor, who then communicates such disclosures to the FDA as part of regulatory filings. Because many sponsors also provide research support, in terms of infrastructure and other equipment, directly to institutions, it is not clear whether a sponsor can properly manage a possible dual financial relationship when a particular investigator is conducting a clinical trial and the investigator's institution also receives support from the sponsor.

Increasingly, journals are requiring disclosure of financial interests for authors submitting manuscripts for publication. It is an open question whether disclosure resolves questions of scientific integrity and whether it helps bolster public trust in the research enterprise.

Infrastructure and Operational Considerations

Because the recommendations in the recent guidance and reports far surpass current regulatory requirements for managing conflicts of interests, institutions wishing to implement policies and procedures in this area may have to consider additional infrastructure and operational investments. Some examples are:

- Information technology to automate the review and updating of financial interests
- Publication of policies and forms online for easier access and for increased public transparency
- Development of educational programs for institutional faculty and staff
- Additional staff, space, and other operational resources for administration of conflict-of-interest review and investigation

All the recent reports and guidance documents are silent on the specifics regarding what sort of compliance monitoring should occur for conflict-of-interest management. Nevertheless, given that the recommended practices exceed the current regulatory requirements, institutions also need to consider additional compliance-monitoring efforts.

Conclusion

Through this analysis of policy-development features for both individual and institutional conflicts of interest, the normative "bottom line," best stated in the DHHS guidance, should remain paramount as institutions and individuals grapple with these issues: "Financial relationships in human research should not compromise any of . . . [the] principles [of the Belmont Report]. Openness and honesty are indicators of respect for persons, characteristics that promote ethical research and can only strengthen the research process" (U.S. Department of Health and Human Services 2003, 15457).

ACKNOWLEDGMENTS

I wish to thank the following individuals who either provided feedback on the manuscript or were instrumental in its development: Michele Russell-Einhorn, J.D.; Rick Rohrbach, M.B.A.; Thomas Puglisi, Ph.D.; and Kim Gunter, J.D., L.L.M. In addition, I thank Erica Rose, J.D., for her commentary on the drafts.

This chapter is based on a combination of two presentations and a published manuscript. "A Comparative Analysis of Selected Guidances on Conflicts of Interest in Biomedical Research," with coauthor Michele Russell-Einhorn, was presented at a meeting of the Hastings Center Project "Ethical Issues in the Management of Financial Conflicts of Interest in Biomedical Research" (funded by the Patrick and Catherine Weldon Donaghue Medical Research Foundation), April 10, 2003. "Conflicts of Interest: Academic and Industry Perspectives" was presented at a meeting of the Society of Research Administrators International, October 24, 2004. The manuscript was published as D. J. Perlman, and M. L. Lester, "Financial Conflicts of Interest in Biomedical Research: An Examination of Current Regulations, Recent Guidance, and Policy Development Considerations," in *Proceedings of the Society of Research Administrators International* (2003 Annual Meeting), 145–62. In its proceedings, the Society of Research Administrators publishes articles from which presentations at its annual meetings are drawn. Due to the limited circulation of these manuscripts to conference registrants, the society encourages authors to publish manuscripts in peer-reviewed journals.

NOTES

1. Not all financial interests are, or result in, conflicts of interest. The term *financial interest* simply represents what bioethicist Thomas Murray (2002) calls "a description of a state of affairs." Only when financial interests affect or appear to affect the collection, analysis, and interpretation of data, scientific objectivity and integrity, and, ultimately, public trust should we ascribe moral or ethical status to such states of affairs as warranting management, reduction, or elimination.

2. I am indebted to Matthew Lester for providing a first draft for some material in the following sections in our previous publication, Perlman and Lester 2003.

3. All of the reports also endorse the recommendation that the IRB should not be the sole locus of authority for management of financial conflicts of interest.

4. The National Institutes of Health Office of Government Ethics issued a recommendation

that all NIH employees be strictly prohibited from entering into consulting arrangements with commercial sponsors (Agres 2004). Soon afterward, the NIH director issued a directive that prevented such arrangements—perhaps illustrating how individual investigators' conflicts of interest, whether perceived or actual, can affect the public's perception of the institution as a whole (U.S. Department of Health and Human Services 2005).

REFERENCES

AAMC Task Force on Financial Conflicts of Interest in Clinical Research. 2001. *Protecting Subjects, Preserving Trust, Promoting Progress: Policy and Guidelines for the Oversight of Individual Financial Interests in Human Subjects Research.* Washington, DC: Association of American Medical Colleges. www.aamc.org.

———. 2002. *Protecting Subjects, Preserving Trust, Promoting Progress II: Principles and Recommendations for Oversight of an Institution's Financial Interests in Human Subjects Research.* Washington, DC: Association of American Medical Colleges. www.aamc.org.

Agres, T. 2004. NIH ethics report draws critics. *The Scientist*, Aug. 12.

Appelbaum, P. S., L. H. Roth, C. W. Lidz, and W. Winslade. 1987. False hopes and best data: Consent to research and the therapeutic misconception. *Hastings Center Report* 17 (2): 20–24.

Association of American Universities Task Force on Research Accountability. 2002. *Report on Individual and Institutional Conflict of Interest.* Washington, DC: Association of American Universities. www.aau.edu.

Coyle, S. L. 2002a. Physician-industry relations. Part I: Individual physicians. *Annals of Internal Medicine* 136 (5): 396–402.

———. 2002b. Physician-industry relations. Part II: Organizational issues. *Annals of Internal Medicine* 136 (5): 403–6.

Drug Information Association. 2004. A question of balance: Medical ethics in clinical trials. *Drug Information Association Forum*, Oct.: 6–8.

Gillis, J. 2002. A hospital's conflict of interest. *Washington Post*, June 30.

International Committee of Medical Journal Editors. 2001. *Publication Ethics: Sponsorship, Authorship, and Accountability.* Philadelphia, PA: International Committee of Medical Journal Editors. www.icmje.org.

Lemonick, M. D., and A. Goldstein. 2002. At your own risk. *Time*, Apr. 14, 159.

Mahoney, J. D. 1999. *NIH Initiative to Reduce Regulatory Burden: Identification of Issues and Potential Solutions.* Washington, DC: Office of Extramural Research, National Institutes of Health. http://grants.nih.gov/grants/policy/policy.htm.

McCluskey, L. F. 2002. Therapeutic misconception/misrepresentation? *PennBioethics* 10 (3): 4–5.

Morin, K., H. Rakatansky, F. A. Riddick, L. J. Morse, J. M. O'Bannon, M. S. Goldrich, P. Ray, M. Weiss, R. M. Sade, and M. A. Spillman. 2002. American Medical Association (AMA) Council on Ethical and Judicial Affairs (CEJA) report: Managing conflicts of interest in the conduct of clinical trials. *JAMA* 287 (1):78–84.

Murray, T. H. 2002. What do we mean by "conflicts of interest?" Paper presented at the first meeting of the Hastings Center Project "Ethical Issues in the Management of Financial

Conflicts of Interest in Research in Health, Medicine and the Biomedical Sciences," Garrison, NY. May.

National Bioethics Advisory Commission. 2001. *Ethical and Policy Issues in Research Involving Human Participants.* Washington, DC: National Bioethics Advisory Commission. http://bioethics.georgetown.edu/nbac/pubs.html.

National Commission for the Protection of Human Subjects in Biomedical and Behavioral Research. 1979. *The Belmont Report: Ethical Principles and Guidelines for the Protection of Human Subjects.* Washington, DC: U.S. Department of Health, Education, and Welfare.

Nelson, R. M. 2001. Protocol 126 and "The Hutch." *IRB: Ethics and Human Research* 23 (3): 14–16.

Perlman, D. J., and M. L. Lester. 2003. Financial conflicts of interest in biomedical research: An examination of current regulations, recent guidance, and policy development considerations. Paper presented at the Proceedings of the Society of Research Administrators International Annual Meeting, Pittsburgh, PA.

Pharmaceutical Research and Manufacturers of America. 2002. *PhRMA Code on Interactions with Healthcare Professionals.* Washington, DC: Pharmaceutical Research and Manufacturers of America. www.phrma.org/publications.

Russell-Einhorn, M. K., and J. T. Puglisi, eds. 2001. *The Institutional Review Board Reference Book: Protecting Those Who Volunteer to Participate in Research.* Washington, DC: Pricewaterhouse Coopers LLP.

U.S. Department of Health and Human Services. 1991. 45 CFR 46.107(e). *Federal Register* 56 (June 18): 28003.

———. 2001. *Draft Interim Guidance "Financial Relationships in Clinical Research: Issues for Institutions, Clinical Investigators, and IRBs to Consider When Dealing with Issues of Financial Interests and Human Subject Protection."* Washington, DC: U.S. Department of Health and Human Services.

———. 2003. Draft "Financial relationships and interests in research involving human subjects: Guidance for human subject protection." *Federal Register* 68 (Mar. 31): 15456–460.

———. 2005. Supplemental standards of ethical conduct and financial disclosure requirements for employees of the Department of Health and Human Services. *Federal Register* 70 (Feb. 3): 5543–65.

U.S. Food and Drug Administration. 1981. 21 CFR 56.107(e). *Federal Register* 46 (Jan. 27): 8975.

———. 1998. 21 CFR Part 54: Financial disclosure by clinical investigators. *Federal Register* 63 (Feb. 2): 5250.

U.S. General Accounting Office. 2001. *Biomedical Research: HHS Direction Needed to Address Financial Conflicts of Interest.* Washington, DC: U.S. General Accounting Office. www.gao.gov.

U.S. Public Health Service. 1995. 42 CFR Part 50, Subpart F: Responsibility of applicants for promoting objectivity in research for which PHS funding is sought. *Federal Register* 60 (July 11): 35815; 60 (July 31): 39076.

CHAPTER 10

Financial Conflicts of Interest in Research with Human Subjects

A Clinical Research Organization's Perspective

DOUGLAS PEDDICORD, PH.D.

The Role of For-Profit Entities in Clinical Trials Research

A subset of clinical research is pursued to facilitate the development and regulatory approval of new drugs and new medical devices. While this research grows out of bench science and basic clinical investigation, which may be initiated by individual scientists, clinical trials are aimed at translating promising laboratory discoveries into improved clinical practice. They take place on a scale that may require tens or hundreds of investigators and research sites and thousands of human subjects. This research is labor-intensive and time-consuming, and the costs can be enormous—as much as $900 million to $1.2 billion or more to develop a single new drug or biologic over a ten- to fifteen-year development cycle (Tufts Center for Study of Drug Development 2003, 2006). Such drug-development costs can be borne only by government or large companies with significant resources.

This chapter examines the role of for-profit entities—commercial sponsors and the organizations with which these sponsors contract—in clinical research with human subjects. It provides a perspective on the different financial conflicts that may occur when for-profit and nonprofit entities conduct clinical trials research and explores the management of such conflicts in each case.

Pharmaceutical and biotechnology companies must conduct clinical trials (i.e., trials in humans) of new diagnostic or therapeutic products. Historically, studies not conducted by the companies themselves were contracted out to academic sites. As recently as 1988, an estimated 80 percent of investigators engaged in clinical trials research worked in academic medical centers (AMCs) (Lightfoot, Sanford, and Shefrin 1999). But within ten years, approximately 60 percent of such investigators were conducting their studies in group practices and other office-based settings (Hovde and Seskin 1997), and today that number is believed to be 70 percent or more. This movement of sponsor-funded clinical trials toward community-based investigators and patient populations accessed through office and clinic settings, rather than through tertiary care medical centers, anticipated a key component of the National Institutes of Health (NIH) Roadmap, proposed in 2003. As NIH director, Elias Zerhouni (2003, 64), said at the time: "Although biomedical research has succeeded in converting many lethal diseases into chronic, treatable conditions, continued success requires that the United States recast its entire system of clinical research . . . Clinical research needs to develop new partnerships among organized patient communities, community-based physicians and academic researchers. In the past, all research for a clinical trial could be conducted in one academic center; that is unlikely to be true in the future."

According to Henderson (2000), for-profit contract research organizations (CROs) administered some 60 percent of the research grant dollars spent by pharmaceutical companies in 2000, compared with the 40 percent of pharmaceutical industry grants made directly to AMCs. Put another way, CROs are involved in about two-thirds of all the clinical trials that are not conducted in-house by pharmaceutical and biotechnology companies. While CROs use many AMC-based investigators, they have facilitated both a significant increase in the number of community-based physicians involved in clinical research and a broadening of practice settings from which clinical trials participants are drawn.

The enormous growth of CRO involvement in clinical trials research has taken place over just twenty years, and today, the industry remains little known, even to most health policymakers. In a seminal article describing the industrialization of clinical research, Rettig (2000) examined various factors underlying the increasing amount of clinical trials work that was contracted out in the preceding decade and fueled the emergence of CROs and other for-profit entities in today's clinical research environment. First and foremost is the search by the commercial sponsors of clinical research for greater efficiency and greater speed in the lengthening development cycle (U.S. Food and Drug Administration 2004). For sponsor companies, outsourcing provides an efficient means of expanding and contracting research capacity to match the ebbs and flows in the development pipeline. And, especially for smaller companies such as emerging biotechnology firms, specialized research organizations furnish the clinical research resources and regulatory expertise necessary to conduct clinical trials, which many young companies lack. Further, many CROs develop research competencies in specific therapeutic areas, and the larger CROs provide a genuinely global reach in terms of investigators, research sites, and potential human subjects.

Contract research organizations provide a wide range of research services, which may include consultation in study design; facilitation of investigator and subject recruitment; initiation of the research site and liaison with the institutional review board (IRB); provision of research staff, including trained study coordinators and monitors; central laboratory and quality assurance services; data management and data analysis; and guidance through the complex regulatory environment. In short, the CRO has emerged as a specialized organization whose primary purpose is to provide the clinical trials research functions needed by commercial sponsors for the development and regulatory approval of new medicines and products, in contrast to (and as an alternative to) the AMC, whose many other missions (including provision of medical care, medical education, and a range of community-specific functions) typically compete with and often significantly encumber the resources devoted to clinical research. As Davidoff et al. (2001, 825) suggested, when it comes to clinical trials, CROs "can do the job for less money and with fewer hassles than academic investigators."

Though the world of clinical research has changed dramatically, then, the importance of the private sector in today's research environment remains overlooked. For instance, a report from the U.S. General Accounting Office (2001, 1) suggested that "responsibility for the protection of human subjects in biomedical research exists at three levels: at the federal level are agencies, such as HHS [U.S. Department of Health and Human Services]; at the institutional level are research institutions, including universities and academic medical centers; and at the individual investigator level are physicians, scientists, and other professionals." Instead of "agencies—institutions—individuals," a more complete list of stakeholders would include, at a minimum, "sponsors—CROs and other providers of contractual services—institutions and institutional review boards (IRBs)—investigators and research site personnel—agencies and regulators—and patients."

Pharmaceutical and other commercial sponsor companies may indeed transfer to a CRO some or all of the regulatory responsibilities for clinical trials as mandated under Food and Drug Administration (FDA) regulations (see 21 Code of Federal Regulations [CFR] Part 54 [U.S. Food and Drug Administration 1998]), but the CRO is not simply a proxy for the sponsor. Rather, in many ways, CROs are hybrid entities, playing a variety of roles with the various stakeholders in the clinical research enterprise. Thus, in relation to some aspects of study conduct and monitoring, the CRO looks like a *sponsor*. Yet, at the same time, the CRO has the characteristics of a *research institution*, if by that we mean an entity that may identify clinical investigators, provide or arrange for dedicated research facilities, conduct any or all phases of the research, and be responsible for regulatory compliance. For the investigator and investigative site, meanwhile, the CRO may be variously a *resource* for regulatory expertise and a hands-on *overseer*, monitoring and auditing the conduct of the clinical trial. In the end, for the sponsor, the investigator, and even the regulator (the FDA), the CRO may be alternately *associate* and *intermediary*—and often it is the only entity that has a real-time overview of all the participants in a given project.

As research and development spending by the pharmaceutical industry has outstripped the research spending of the NIH, concerns have grown that the motivation to develop new and profitable products may bias the conduct and reporting of clinical trials research, particularly where such research is conducted using pharmaceutical industry money or with the involvement of a CRO. For instance, the Hastings Center research project that led to this volume aims to pay "special attention to the ethical implications of the role of private for-profit corporations in the financing and execution of research" (Murray et al., 2002–3, 1). Some authors (e.g., Relman and Angell 2002) go as far as to argue that while pharmaceutical companies and other commercial sponsors should pay for clinical trials, they should have no say in the design and conduct of the trials or in the collection, analysis, and interpretation of the data, and that "hired businesses" that conduct clinical trials for the drug companies should be eliminated.

While the potential for financial and other conflicts of interest should be guarded against in all research, the assumption that the pursuit of profit and the progress of science and medicine must inherently conflict deserves examination. For instance, the obligation of "industry-sponsored" investigators to produce accurate findings in a timely manner within the constraints of an agreed-upon budget may exert no greater pressures (and potential for bias) than those felt by investigators whose grant support (and professional aspirations) has them striving for publications, tenure, and additional grants. And, in reality, the marketplace is a powerful guardian of behavior for companies conducting clinical research on contract. In general, CROs have little revenue that is not directly related to the conduct of research; they do not hold patents, are not eligible for federal grants, and have no endowments. A CRO with a poor safety record, for instance, will quickly lose business to its competitors and lose value as a company. There is little empirical evidence for the presumption that scientific integrity and ethical behavior are solely the province of the academy—or of government, for that matter.

Because CROs provide services to pharmaceutical and other sponsors on a contractual basis, some critics believe that these organizations are interested only in positive research outcomes. In fact, the contractual obligations of the CRO are to implement and manage a clinical trial in accordance with the study protocol, to ensure the quality and integrity of the research data, and to ensure compliance with FDA and other, international regulations. The contract between pharmaceutical research sponsor and CRO stipulates the research services to be rendered, without regard to the specific results of any given study, and never requires that the CRO produce positive (or negative, for that matter) research findings.

Actual and Potential Financial Conflicts in Clinical Trials Research

In March 2003, the U.S. Department of Health and Human Services (DHHS) published a draft document entitled "Financial Relationships and Interests in Research involving Human Subjects: Guidance for Human Subject Protection." The document suggested that "a financial interest related to a research study may be a conflicting financial interest if it will, or may be reasonably expected to, create a bias stemming from that financial interest" (15457). To operationalize this definition to all the participants involved in the funding and conduct of clinical trials research, in this chapter I define a financial conflict as financial or related considerations that may color the design, review, approval, conduct, monitoring, analysis, or reporting of research conducted by or under the auspices of an individual, institution, or other for-profit or nonprofit entity.

Any of the stakeholders in a clinical study, including the sponsor, the IRB, the CRO or other provider of contractual services, the AMC, or the investigator, may be biased by financial considerations. And within each of these broad categories of stakeholder, a number of individuals may experience significant pressure as a result of financial interests that could bias the conduct and reporting of the research. For instance, principal investigators rely heavily on the performance of study staff; the CRO depends on the research expertise and ethical integrity of study monitors and auditors; and the institution-based IRB counts on resources provided by organizations that are often under enormous financial strains—and in each instance, the performance of individuals "on the line" with regard to the recognition and management of actual or potential financial conflicts is likely to reflect the culture and circumstances of the larger entity.

So, what are examples of the kinds of financial consideration that might cause bias at the level of the investigator or research organization (AMC or CRO)?

- First and foremost are direct payments or other compensation that are significantly in excess of the actual costs of the research; whether this is called investigational site "profit" or academic institution "overhead," such compensation may create a biasing financial interest for the investigator or research organization.
- Less common, perhaps, are increased equity, interest, or other non-cash reward as a result of research study findings—for example, increased value of existing stock holdings, or the granting of increased equity or other financial interest in the sponsor company, or the potential for patent and licensing interests.
- Finally, the least immediately rewarding (and potentially biasing) financial consideration is the future value of new grants and contracts that may be awarded to the investigator, AMC, CRO, or other research entity, based on the results of a study or set of studies.

For the investigator or research organization or institution, potentially biasing financial interests may be derived from private sector or nonprofit funding sources—that is, compensation for research services that is "excessive" or beyond fair market value, increased financial or intellectual property interests, or the promise of repeat "business" all can be provided by federal dollars as well as by funding from for-profit entities, as anyone familiar with stories of Pentagon purchasing of $800 toilet seats can appreciate. Yet, in clinical research, policymakers and legislators (see Kennedy 2002) often seem to proceed from the premise that federal or other nonprofit funding cannot corrupt, whereas pharmaceutical company dollars are, somehow, inherently conflicted and biasing. In reality, potential financial conflicts of interest, whether occurring in CROs, AMCs, or any other research entities, should be scrutinized in the same manner and to the same degree whether the source of the research funding is a federal agency, a nonprofit organization, or a for-profit corporation.

Existing regulations governing investigators' financial interests and potential financial conflicts of interest treat federally funded research conducted under the Common Rule differently from commercially sponsored clinical trials research, which is subject to FDA regulations. Under the Common Rule, an investigator reports any significant financial interest—defined as an amount exceeding $10,000—to his or her institution. The research institution must then provide an assurance to the DHHS secretary that it has in place an administrative process to identify financial interests and will report any financial interests that it has determined "could directly and significantly affect" the research ("but not the nature of the interest or other details") (see 45 CFR Part 94 and 42 CFR Part 50, Subpart F [U.S. Public Health Service 1995a, 1995b]), along with how conflicting interests will be managed, reduced, or eliminated (see also Public Health Service Act of 2004, 42 United States Code Sec. 493A, "Protection against Financial Conflicts of Interest in Certain Projects of Research," 571). Meanwhile, for clinical research regulated by the FDA (see 21 CFR Part 54) the investigator must disclose to the sponsor (or CRO) whether he or she has any financial interest in the success or failure of the study; has received any payments from the sponsor greater than $25,000 in the past two years, other than for study-related costs; or holds an interest in a sponsor's stock of greater than $50,000 or in stock of another company that would significantly benefit by the study. Later, the sponsor must provide to the FDA a list of all clinical investigators involved in clinical trials studies that are submitted to the agency for review and must, for each investigator, either disclose financial arrangements that may be conflicting or certify the absence of such a financial conflict.

In brief, investigators involved in FDA-regulated research certify to the sponsor the absence of significant financial interest or disclose such an interest, whereas federally funded investigators report any significant financial interests to their institution, which then must "manage, reduce or eliminate" any conflicts of interest it has determined to be significant and report on those efforts to the funding source. These two approaches reflect the differences between the "assurance" model of regulation and oversight of the Common Rule and the strict "compliance" model of FDA regulation. Under Public

Health Service Act regulations, investigators and their institutions "assure" the federal government that they have considered the potential effect of a significant financial interest, but the locus for the determination of the "rebuttable assumption" regarding the existence of an actual conflict rests with the institution (i.e., the AMC or other entity), not with the federal funding agency. Under FDA-regulated research, by contrast, the investigator's disclosure is made to the sponsor, and while the sponsor has some latitude in determining whether certain financial arrangements with investigators could introduce bias, the sponsor is not given the opportunity to "manage, reduce or eliminate" financial conflicts on its own but must report either the presence or absence of potentially conflicting financial arrangements to the regulator (the FDA).

Undoubtedly, both commercial research sponsors and AMCs and other research institutions are subject to shorter- and longer-term opportunities for financial gain that "may color" the conduct and reporting of a research study. But the potential consequences of their decision-making on significant financial interests that could affect the integrity of any given study are quite different. Under the Public Health Service Act, the DHHS secretary may require that a research institution disclose the existence of any financial interest in "each public presentation" of the results of a funded project, an action that is meant to increase the transparency of financial interests. But the FDA "may consider clinical studies inadequate and the data inadequate if, among other things, appropriate steps have not been taken in the design, conduct, reporting and analysis of the studies to minimize bias" (see 21 CFR Sec. 54.1[b]). At such a point, the agency may initiate an audit of the study data, request further data analyses to evaluate the effect of individual investigators' data on the study outcome, or refuse to accept the study results as a basis for FDA approval of a new product. In contrast to the "transparency" of financial interest (and potential for conflict) engendered by the Public Health Service approach, the ultimate sanction for commercially sponsored clinical research subject to FDA regulation is a "data death penalty." In the for-profit world, the economic implications of a delay caused by the use of an investigator who has a financial conflict are generally extremely persuasive and will cause the sponsor to avoid the investigator altogether.

If the potential consequences of an investigator's financial conflict differ, depending on the source of funding for a clinical study (i.e., whether conducted with a grant from a federal agency or a contract from a commercial sponsor), the mechanism of oversight is in some ways similar, regardless of where the research is conducted. That is, in most instances, the principal overseeing entity is directly "in the path" of the financial conflict and has its own financial interest in the study. For example, if the study is conducted at an AMC, the initial assessment of any potential conflict is likely to be handled by its IRB or its conflict-of-interest committee (AAMC Taskforce on Financial Conflicts of Interest in Clinical Research 2002). But both the IRB and the conflict-of-interest committee are part of the very institution at which the study is being conducted—an institution that clearly has a financial interest in the study in question because it is part of the institution's research portfolio and funding stream. Meanwhile, if the study takes place in a community-based hospital or practice (or other non-AMC setting) under FDA regulations, it is up to the sponsor, which clearly has a financial interest in the outcome of the study, to ensure that the investigator does not have a conflict of interest. In effect, except when an independent (commercial) IRB—which does not have either a short-term or long-term financial interest in the *outcome* of a given study—delves into an investigator's potential financial conflict of interest, the initial layer of oversight deployed by research institutions and research companies is encumbered by greater or lesser degrees of self-interest.

Pharmaceutical companies, however, in constructing financial arrangements with clinical investigators, are guided by voluntary industry standards designed to prevent bias due to excessive compensation. Basic principles of financial compensation articulated by the Pharmaceutical Research and Manufacturers of America (2002, revised 2009, 15) stipulate that "payment to clinical investigators or their institutions should be reasonable and based on work performed by the investigator and the investigator's staff, not on any other considerations." Elaborated further, these for-profit companies say that payment or compensation of any sort cannot be tied to the outcome of a clinical trial; that the investigator and his or her immediate family should not have any ownership interest in the specific product being studied; that investigators and institutions should not be compensated in stock or stock options; and that incentives that may cause investigators to coerce patient participation should not be used.

If compensation is to be reasonable and based on work performed, then the creation of the clinical study budget is key to managing the potential for investigators' financial conflicts of interest. Ideally, the clinical study budget should reflect every cost associated with the conduct of a clinical trial, from salaries, operating costs, and overhead to IRB review and adverse-event management. In the for-profit world, it is axiomatic that a contract with an investigator should specify services to be performed and have deliverables. The sponsor (or CRO) must develop a process for determining the "fair market value" of services, such as per-procedure costs, physician time, study coordinator time, advertising and other recruitment costs, and the like. A sponsor or CRO may develop an overhead cost calculation for each research site or type of study or, for most studies, may apply a standard overhead cost rate.

If the primary objective of the clinical study budget is to create a fair and explicit contractual relationship between the sponsor and the investigator or institution, its secondary purpose should be to establish transparency in the funding stream—because without some possibility of "following the money," it is difficult to see how any entity, whether IRB, conflict-of-interest committee, or regulator, can fully understand the investigator's or institution's financial interest in the clinical trial. Unfortunately, federal funding mechanisms do not encourage such transparency, as grants pay indirect (overhead) costs that vary enormously across research institutions, ranging from 30 percent to nearly 100 percent of the direct costs incurred to conduct the study. (Meanwhile, an article in *CenterWatch* estimated overhead costs of 17% in non-academic settings [Borfitz 2003], suggesting that considerable additional "profit" to the institution is built into the indirect cost component of federal grants.) The federal government certainly has a legitimate interest in broadly funding the research mission of the nation's AMCs, but when as much as half of total grant funding flows not to the cost of a specific study but to support the institution in general, it becomes unclear how an entity within that institution, such as the IRB or conflict-of-interest committee, can accurately tease out the financial interest (and potential financial conflict of interest) of the investigator or the institution with regard to the grant funding a particular study. This issue is illustrated by a comment from the director of clinical research practices at a leading AMC: "why do a pharmaceutical company study with [a] 25% indirect rate when you could do a federally funded study at a 57% indirect rate?" (CenterWatch 2003, 12).

Even as there are concerns that investigators and institutions are pursuing "too many dollars" in the clinical research arena, many factors constrain adequate budgeting of clinical trials, and some reports indicate that both AMCs and community-based and other research sites are reconsidering the fiscal viability of clinical research participation. For instance, "Although most sites report that they are generating a 10% to 12% annual profit [in commercially sponsored trials], recent data suggest that sites may be operating closer to breaking even when 'hidden' or uncompensated costs are accounted for" (Borfitz 2003, 1). And Dr. David Korn, senior vice-president of the Association of American Medical Colleges, stated in a study group discussion that research grants to AMCs are insufficient to cover the full costs of research and that AMCs "lose 10 to 30 cents on every [research] dollar" (Hastings Center Project, Work Group, Apr. 11, 2003). In the for-profit world, downward pressures on clinical trials budgets include the facts that the core pricing for research services, beyond per-procedure costs, remains relatively flat and inflation is typically not figured into the investigator's grant contract. Simply, when it comes to conflicts of interest that may be engendered by the financing of clinical trials research, the problems observed may more often reflect the reality of "too few dollars" being allocated to a given study than the pursuit of excessive "profit" by the investigator or institution.

One potential effect of inadequate study budgeting is an erosion of performance at the research site. That is, if the research budget is not clearly structured to ensure that investigators and institutions are fairly compensated for efforts to conduct a study of high quality and consistent with reasonable timelines, then experience in the for-profit world suggests that more funds will need to be spent on remediation, including monitoring for enrollment and protocol violations and data queries and corrections. The interaction between budgeting and performance is sometimes illustrated when investigators take on overlapping studies in their therapeutic area of expertise and subsequently devote greater attention to whichever study is "paying the most." In every instance, the investigator and all the other participants, whether sponsor, CRO, AMC, or IRB, should be aware of the amount of financial, clinical, regulatory, and other resources needed to perform the study properly—and a fair and detailed study budget is an important mechanism for reducing the likelihood that financial interests will adversely affect the conduct of the study.

Before leaving this discussion of study budgeting, two additional issues deserve mention. First, there has been controversy over the use of financial incentives by some sponsor companies to "motivate" investigators to encourage volunteer enrollment, which is often the most difficult aspect of a clinical trial. Even when such payment is structured to reinforce strong enrollment performance rather than elicit improved effort by poorly performing research sites, sponsors and CROs are aware that such an incentive may create both the potential for and the appearance of a financial interest that could bias the study. On this matter, the Pharmaceutical and Research Manufacturers of

America's principles (2002, revised 2009, 15) state that "when enrollment is particularly challenging, reasonable additional payments may be made to compensate the clinical investigator or institution for time and effort spent on extra recruiting efforts to enroll appropriate research participants."

Second, in terms of evaluating whether a clinical study budget is likely to increase or decrease the chances of a financial bias that may color the conduct of a clinical trial, an issue arises from the very different construction of budgets by for-profit and nonprofit sponsors of research. To illustrate: DHHS, in its draft guidance on financial relationships and interests in research involving human subjects (U.S. Department of Health and Human Services 2003, 15459) suggested that IRBs and others looking at actual or potential financial conflicts should ask whether individuals or institutions involved in the research "receive payment per participant . . . and are those payments within the norm?" In a comment on this guidance, the Association of Clinical Research Organizations (2003, 3), a group of leading CROs, remarked that "calculation of study budgets based on per participant costs is a standard practice in commercially-sponsored research. Simply, sponsors of FDA-regulated studies rarely, if ever, provide a total upfront grant for an estimated number of subjects, as may occur with NIH and other federal grants. Further, the use of per participant budgeting provides a level of transparency regarding the financing of a study that is far better than that offered by the direct costs–indirect cost rate (including institution 'facilities and administration') grant model used for federally-funded studies." Just as existing regulations (see 45 CFR and 21 CFR) alternately take an "assurance" or "compliance" approach to the disclosure and management of potential financial interests and conflicts, so, too, the "apples" and "oranges" of federal and commercial sponsor budgeting makes meaningful comparisons of investigators' and institutions' financial interests (and potential conflicts) hard to come by.

Conclusion

In a world where dollars are dollars, the assumption that an investigator's or research institution's clinical study funding is somehow fundamentally different if it is received from a "financially interested" entity (meaning an entity, such as a pharmaceutical company, whose financial interests would reasonably seem to be affected by the conduct or outcome of a project), rather than from federal or nonprofit entities with no clear financial stake (but, of course, with other levels of "investment" in the success of the project), does not appear reasonable. That is, distinguishing between federal or other non-profit dollars and "for-profit" dollars is not likely to be useful in understanding whether a clinical researcher is or is not bringing in funding to his or her practice or institution and thus should be considered a rainmaker or a liability, with the attendant potential for financial conflict associated with each status. Whether in an academic medical center or in a for-profit setting, the real issue for the individual investigator is whether payments (or other financial inducements, such as patent or stock interests) received or promised are in excess of the reasonable costs of the study and therefore "may color" the conduct or reporting of the clinical trial.

From this perspective, proposals for legislation (see Kennedy 2002) or regulation that would exempt salary or payments for research services when such payments are made "by or through" a nonprofit entity, such as an AMC, serve more to obscure than to control potential financial conflicts. Again, at the investigator level, the locus of the potential financial conflict lies in the "contractual" relationship between the funding source and the investigator. And it is entirely reasonable that others, from institutions and IRBs to CROs and conflict-of-interest committees, should be involved in evaluating and monitoring that relationship. But to interpose one of those other entities, such as the conflict-of-interest committee, as the sole arbiter of potential financial conflict only shifts the locus of the potential conflict from investigator to institution and, in practice, continues the current differing approaches to the identification and management of financial conflicts based on the source of funding. Such an approach does not contribute to the improvement of human subjects protections, regardless of where the clinical trial is to be conducted.

Because both the "assurance" and "compliance" models have strengths and weaknesses, some observers have advocated a combined model—an approach that seeks to "trust but verify." For example, if existing regulations (45 CFR and 21 CFR) were harmonized, then investigators' financial disclosure would always be obtained upfront (as is true today) and be subject to review by the institution (45 CFR) and the sponsor (21 CFR). If a nonprofit funding source, such as the NIH, also undertook a review of the potential for financial conflict at the investigator level, and the IRB did as well, then the matrix of responsibility would extend to include all the players. That is, the determination that a given investigator holds a significant financial interest likely to induce an actual or potential financial conflict of interest and, therefore, should not conduct a specific study would be a responsibility shared jointly by the funding source (whether for-profit or nonprofit), the IRB, and the "institution" (whether AMC or CRO)—and not, as is the case today, a responsibility held solely by the institution or the sponsor, each of which may have considerable financial or other interests in the clinical research.

Consistent and uniform oversight of actual and potential financial conflicts would be facilitated further by significantly increasing the transparency of funding mechanisms and by encouraging disclosure of financial interests to human subjects (e.g., "Clinical investigators are encouraged to disclose to potential research participants during the informed consent process that the investigator and/or the institution is receiving payment for the conduct of the clinical trial" [Pharmaceutical and Research Manufacturers of America 2002, revised 2009]). And the same requirements for the disclosure, review, and management of actual and potential financial conflicts of interest should apply to all clinical trials research, regardless of the source of funding or the site where the research is conducted.

Despite what some might suggest, financial conflicts are not ubiquitous in clinical trials research funded by pharmaceutical, biotechnology, and other commercial companies. Neither is there evidence that the site where the clinical trial is conducted—whether academic medical center or community hospital or private medical practice—can be used to characterize the likelihood of bias in the conduct of the research. This is not to argue that there have not been instances of financial conflicts of interest linked to bias in clinical trials research funded by for-profit companies, but rather to point out that financial interests can and do have a negative influence on the conduct of clinical research whether the funding comes from the federal government (Wilson and Heath 2001) or from a for-profit entity, and whether the research took place in a nonprofit institution (e.g., Weiss and Nelson 1999), a government site (e.g., Pear 2003), or a for-profit setting. While intuitively plausible, the notion that the role of private for-profit corporations in the financing and execution of research brings unique or increased dangers of conflict and bias into the research enterprise is an assumption only, and one that ignores significant countervailing influences on the profit motive in the conduct of clinical research, including a high degree of public scrutiny. In fact, it is equally plausible to suggest that, rather than bringing unique or increased dangers, the for-profit "marketplace" brings to clinical research better quality and less tolerance for shoddy performance or misapplied energies than does the largely self-regulated and self-contained world of the scientific "academy." (For a view of the deleterious effects of "in-house" oversight of research, see, for example, *Grimes v. Kennedy Krieger Institute, Inc. et al.*, 366 MD 29, 782 A.2d 807 [Md. Ct. App. 2001].)

In its draft guidance (March 2003), which has since been finalized (May 2004), the DHHS stated:

> Concerns have grown that financial conflicts of interest in research, derived from financial relationships and the financial interests they create, may affect the rights and welfare of human research subjects. Financial interests are not prohibited, and not all financial interests cause conflicts of interest or harm to human subjects. HHS recognizes the complexity of the relationships between government, academia, industry and others, and recognizes that these relationships often legitimately include financial relationships. However, to the extent financial interests may affect the rights and welfare of human subjects in research, IRBs, institutions, and investigators need to consider what actions regarding financial interests may be necessary to protect those subjects. (U.S. Department of Health and Human Services 2004, 26395).

It is important to point out, again, that to the list of "IRBs, institutions, and investigators" it is essential to add "sponsors, CROs, and other providers of contractual services," and this formulation provides an even-handed framing of the issues—one that does not divide the world into "conflicted" dollars and "nonconflicted" dollars or into "acceptable" and "nonacceptable" research sites. The DHHS has focused on the protection of human subjects, and from the perspective of the CRO industry, the same set of financial conflict-of-interest requirements and the same level of oversight should apply to all clinical trials research, regardless of the source of funding or the site where the research is conducted. We suggest that all participants in the research environment develop a fuller awareness of the impact, or potential impact, of financial interests and relationships on the rights and welfare of human subjects.

ACKNOWLEDGMENT

The author is executive director of the Association of Clinical Research Organizations, a trade group that represents the clinical research industry before legislative and regulatory bodies in the United States and other countries. Clinical research organizations assist pharmaceutical, biotechnology, and medical device companies with the conduct of thousands of clinical trials each year and are a key participant in the development of new drugs and new treatments. ACRO member companies employ more than seventy thousand people worldwide and conduct research in more than 115 countries. The views expressed in this chapter are D. Peddicord's and do not represent ACRO policy.

REFERENCES

AAMC Task Force on Financial Conflicts of Interest in Clinical Research. 2002. *Protecting Subjects, Preserving Trust, Promoting Progress II: Principles and Recommendations for Oversight of an Institution's Financial Interests in Human Subjects Research.* Washington, DC: Association of American Medical Colleges.

Association of Clinical Research Organizations. 2003. Comment on draft "Financial Relationships and Interests in Research Involving Human Subjects: Guidance for Human Subject Protection." Docket no. 02N-0475, May 21, 1–3. Washington, DC: Association of Clinical Research Organizations.

Borfitz, D. 2003. Unveiling "hidden costs" in clinical trials. *CenterWatch* 10 (9): 4–8.

CenterWatch. 2003. AHCs face a tightening NIH funding supply. *CenterWatch* 10 (8): 1, 9–14.

Davidoff, F., C. D. DeAngelis, J. M. Drazen, J. Hoey, L. Højgaard, R. Horton, S. Kotzin, et al. 2001. Sponsorship, authorship, and accountability. *New England Journal of Medicine* 345 (11):825–27.

Henderson, L. 2000. More AMCs finding growth from reform. *CenterWatch* 7 (6): 1, 10–13.

Hovde, M., and R. Seskin. 1997. Selecting U.S. clinical investigators. *Applied Clinical Trials,* Feb.: 34–42.

Kennedy, E. 2002. Research Revitalization Act. S. 3060. 107th Congress. Washington, DC: U.S. Senate.

Lightfoot, G. D., S. M. Sanford, and A. P. Shefrin. 1999. Can investigator certification improve the quality of clinical research? *The Monitor,* Fall: 17–21.

Murray T., D. Callahan, M. A. Baily, A. Wasunna, and J. Johnston. 2002–3. Hastings Center Project "Ethical Issues in the Management of Financial Conflicts of Interest in Health and Medical Research." Garrison, NY: Hastings Center.

Pear, R. 2003. U.S. to review research at hospitals for veterans. *New York Times,* Apr. 13.

Pharmaceutical Research and Manufacturers of America. 2002, revised 2009. *Principles on Conduct of Clinical Trials and Communication of Clinical Trial Results.* Washington, DC: Pharmaceutical Research and Manufacturers of America.

Relman, A., and M. Angell. 2002. America's other drug problem. *New Republic,* Dec. 16: 27–41.

Rettig, R. 2000. The industrialization of clinical research. *Health Affairs* 19 (2): 129–46.

Tufts Center for Study of Drug Development. 2003. Post-approval R&D raises total drug development costs to $897 million. *Impact Report* 5 (3): 1–4.

———. 2006. Cost to develop new biotech products is estimated to average $1.2 billion. *Impact Report* 8 (6): 1–3.

U.S. Department of Health and Human Services. 2003. Draft " Financial relationships and interests in research involving human subjects: Guidance for human subject protection." *Federal Register* 68 (61): 15456–60.

———. 2004. Financial relationships and interests in research involving human subjects: Guidance for human subject protection. *Federal Register* 69 (92): 26393–97.

U.S. Food and Drug Administration. 1998. 21 CFR Part 54: Financial disclosure by clinical investigators. *Federal Register* 63 (Feb. 2): 5233–54.

———. 2004. *Innovation or Stagnation? Challenge and Opportunity on the Critical Path to New Medical Products.* Washington, DC: U.S. Food and Drug Administration.

U.S. General Accounting Office. 2001. *Human Subjects Research: HHS Takes Steps to Strengthen Protections, But Concerns Remain.* GAO-01-775T. Washington, DC: U.S. General Accounting Office. 2001.

U.S. Public Health Service. 1995a. 42 CFR Part 50, Subpart F: Responsibility of applicants for promoting objectivity in research for which PHS funding is sought. *Federal Register* 60 (July 11): 180–83.

———. 1995b. 45 CFR Part 94: Conflicts of interest; government contracts. *Federal Register* 60 (July 11): 35817; 60 (July 31): 39076.

Weiss, R., and D. Nelson. 1999. Gene therapy's troubling crossroads: A death raises questions of ethics, profit, science. *Washington Post*, Dec. 31.

Wilson, D., and D. Heath. 2001. Uninformed consent. *Seattle Times*, Mar.

Zerhouni, E. 2003. The NIH Roadmap. *Science* 302 (5642): 63–72.

Index

Page numbers in *italics* refer to figures and tables.

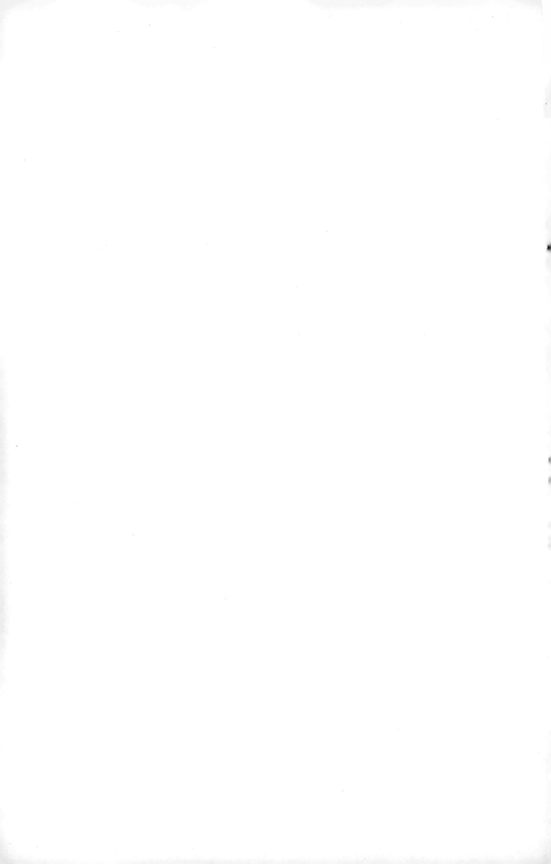